THE
LAP-BAND®
SIMPLIFIED

Frederick M. Tiesenga M.D., FACS

I would like to thank my parents Marvin and Ardythe Tiesenga. My dad was a surgical giant and pioneer in bariatric surgery that I was lucky enough to operate with for years and my mother was a constant, steady force in my life. And to my wife Juce and kids Austin, Hannah and Jen.

ABOUT THE AUTHOR

Dr. Tiesenga is an award-winning board-certified bariatric surgeon who is passionate about helping individuals achieve a healthier lifestyle. He is highly regarded in the field of bariatric surgery and is a Center of Excellence certified surgeon. He is also an affiliate surgeon of the American Society of Bariatric Surgeons. Dr. Tiesenga trains surgeons from around the world to perform bariatric surgery.

DISCLAIMER

The information provided in this book is for informational purposes only and the reader should not use this information as medical care or medical advice. The information in this book is not meant to be a replacement for medical advice given by your physician or medical staff. It is the reader's responsibility to evaluate all information provided in this book and should never use this information to treat, diagnose, or cure any medical or health condition. West Adaptive (publisher), Dr. Frederick Tiesenga, and any related members, managers, officers, employees, consultants, and representatives who were involved in writing, editing and publishing the book disclaim all responsibility for any loss, liability, or risk (personal or otherwise) that incurred (directly or indirectly) from the information that contained in this book. We are also not responsible for any errors, omissions, and inaccuracies from the information provided. By continuing to read this book, the reader indicates that he or she accepts the terms of this disclaimer.

The LAP-BAND® is a trademark of Apollo Endosurgery, Inc. Any third-party trademarks used herein are the property of their respective owners.

Contents

CHAPTER 6. THE FIRST STEPS: PREPARING FOR BARIATRIC SURGERY

CHAPTER 7. WHAT TO EXPECT BEFORE LAP-BAND PROCEDURE?

Chapter 1. Obesity: A Growing Epidemic Gone Global

What Exactly Is Obesity?

To better understand the epidemic of obesity, let's first define what exactly is obesity. Obesity is a disease in which the excess body fat impairs the individual's health.

The U.S. Department of Health and Human Services (HHS), and the World Health Organization (WHO) have both acknowledged that obesity is a disease. Obesity is considered a disease because it can negatively affect you on both physical and psychological levels. In other words, it makes us sick. Excessive weight has been associated with chronic illnesses such as type II diabetes, hypertension, depression, and mobility difficulties just to name a few. What is more shocking, is the statistic from the National Institute of Health (NIH) states that obesity is the second leading cause of preventable death in the USA, right behind tobacco use. In fact, obesity has been labeled as a global epidemic as it is now common in many parts of the world[1].

Why Is Obesity Labeled as an Epidemic?

More than 2 in 3 adults in the United States are considered overweight or have obesity and 1 in 3 adults are obese[2]. This leaves less than a third of the American population to be considered normal weight. These statistics fit the definition of an epidemic as a widespread occurrence of a disease. The United States is not the only country that has been plagued with widespread obesity, other countries have also reported the alarming growth in obesity among their population. In 2016, it was estimated that over 650 million adults worldwide were obese[3]. Some experts have even changed the definition of obesity from epidemic to a pandemic of global proportions.

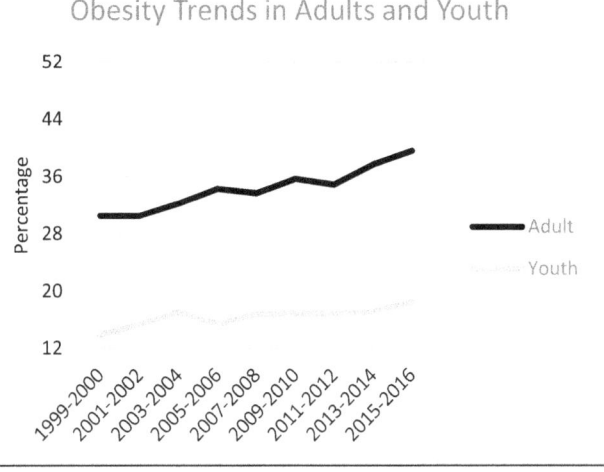

Figure 1: Obesity Trends in Adults (over the age of 20) and Youth (2-19 years old). Data source: NCHS, National Health and Nutrition Examination Survey, 1999-2016.

An Overview of the Global Problem of Obesity

Worldwide obesity has almost tripled in the last four decades. Almost every country in the WHO data repository has experienced an increase in adult obesity from 2010 to 2016. For example, over 31% of the Bahamas' adult population and over 27% of the United Kingdom's population is estimated to be obese[4]. It is also interesting to note that industrial countries are not the only ones that are facing this epidemic, developing countries as well are facing an exploding increase in obesity[5]. In some developing nations such as Gambia, they associate obesity with wealth and beauty, which only further spreads this epidemic[6].

The Factors That Cause Obesity and Weight Gain

The most basic way to explain weight gain: the amount of energy intake is higher than the amount of energy being used. Energy is typically calculated in terms of calories. The human body can store excess energy in adipose tissue, also known as fat. The two common ways accelerated obesity to become an epidemic are:

❖ Increased consumption in calorie-dense foods that are high in fats or sugars.

❖ Decreased physical activity due to changes in the environment in which a sedentary lifestyle is becoming more common.

The modern evolution in food accessibility, transportation, lifestyle and societal changes have made it easier than ever to gain the extra pounds. We are now threatened by cheap and easy to access foods that are high in fats, carbohydrates and sugars. These types of foods make it a much more attractive alternative to healthy choices. Increased access to smartphones, computers and other modern technology create a more sedentary lifestyle making it more difficult to burn off the excess calories.

In today's technologically advanced age, it is possible to order groceries, fully cooked meals, everyday household items and possibly anything else you can think of with a click of a mouse. Leaving your home is now optional and anything you need can be delivered right to your door. It is no longer necessary to go to the store to pick up your daily necessities.

How Exactly Do We Burn Calories?

We burn calories in mainly three ways.

1) **Physical Activity** in addition to your normal daily movements. Examples can include brisk walking, running, swimming, playing sports, and gardening just to name a few. The more active you are, the more calories you will burn. Sitting around all day will burn almost no extra calories outside of your metabolism.

2) **Your Metabolism**, also known as your basal metabolic rate (BMR), is the calories burned without doing anything. Think of it as the calories

required for you to survive, pump blood throughout the body, breathe, and other important bodily functions. Your BMR will differ based on your age, gender, height, and weight. Obese individuals may have a higher BMR compared to a normal weight person due to the extra weight they have to carry, but not by much. Fat tissue just sits there and does not do much to burn calories. Losing weight will result in a lower BMR, meaning the more weight you lose, the fewer calories you will need to survive.

3) **Thermic Effect of Food (TEF)** is the amount of energy necessary to digest the food we eat. On average, it is about 10% of the total calorie intake. For example, if you are on a 1500 calorie diet, your thermic effect of food may be somewhere around 150 calories. We can't really change the way we burn calories due to TEF as the energy expenditure is directly proportional to the amount of calories we intake.

Body Mass Index (BMI) – The Simplest Way to Measure Obesity

Body Mass Index, commonly referred to as BMI, is the most popular and easiest way doctors measure obesity. Measuring your body weight is not accurate enough to gauge weight loss progress. BMI considers not only the body weight but also the height of the individual. A taller person, on average, will weigh more than a shorter one. That is why your height is measured when calculating the BMI to provide more accurate data. Here is how BMI is calculated:

$$BMI = \frac{Your\ Weight\ (lbs.)}{[Your\ Height\ (in.)]^2} \times 703$$

We have included a BMI table on the following pages for your convenience.

How to Use the BMI Table?

Find your height and weight in the BMI chart and then use your finger to trace up to the BMI row to see your approximate BMI. If you do not see your weight on the BMI chart, you can Google "BMI calculator" online to get your current BMI.

Normal Weight: BMI 18.5 to 24.9								
BMI	19	20	21	22	23	24	25	26	27
Height (In.)	Weight (lbs.)								
5' 0"	97	102	107	112	118	123	128	133	138
5' 1"	100	106	111	116	122	127	132	137	143
5' 2"	104	109	115	120	126	131	136	142	147
5' 3"	107	113	118	124	130	135	141	146	152
5' 4"	110	116	122	128	134	140	145	151	157
5' 5"	114	120	126	132	138	144	150	156	162
5' 6"	118	124	130	136	142	148	155	161	167
5' 7"	121	127	134	140	146	153	159	166	172
5' 8"	125	131	138	144	151	158	164	171	177
5' 9"	128	135	142	149	155	162	169	176	182
5' 10"	132	139	146	153	160	167	174	181	188
5' 11"	136	143	150	157	165	172	179	186	193
6' 0"	140	147	154	162	169	177	184	191	199
6' 1"	144	151	159	166	174	182	189	197	204
6' 2"	148	155	163	171	179	186	194	202	210
6' 3"	152	160	168	176	184	192	200	208	216
6' 4"	156	164	172	180	189	197	205	213	221
6' 5"	160	169	177	185	194	202	211	219	228
6' 6"	164	173	182	190	199	208	216	225	234

Table 1.i.: Body Mass Index Table for BMI 19-27

Normal Weight: BMI 18.5 to 24.9								
BMI	28	29	30	31	32	33	34	35	36
Height (In.)	Weight (lbs.)								
5' 0"	143	148	153	158	163	168	174	179	184
5' 1"	148	153	158	164	169	174	180	185	190
5' 2"	153	158	164	169	175	180	186	191	196
5' 3"	158	163	169	175	180	186	191	197	203
5' 4"	163	169	174	180	186	192	197	204	209
5' 5"	168	174	180	186	192	198	204	210	216
5' 6"	173	179	186	192	198	204	210	216	223
5' 7"	178	185	191	198	204	211	217	223	230
5' 8"	184	190	197	203	210	216	223	230	236
5' 9"	189	196	203	209	216	223	230	236	243
5' 10"	195	202	209	216	222	229	236	243	250
5' 11"	200	208	215	222	229	236	243	250	257
6' 0"	206	213	221	228	235	242	250	258	265
6' 1"	212	219	227	235	242	250	257	265	272
6' 2"	218	225	233	241	249	256	264	272	280
6' 3"	224	232	240	248	256	264	272	279	287
6' 4"	230	238	246	254	263	271	279	287	295
6' 5"	236	244	253	261	270	278	287	295	304
6' 6"	242	251	260	268	277	285	294	303	311

Table 1.ii.: Body Mass Index Table for BMI 28-36

Normal Weight: BMI 18.5 to 24.9								
BMI	**37**	**38**	**39**	**40**	**41**	**42**	**43**	**44**	**45**
Height (In.)	Weight (lbs.)								
5′ 0″	189	194	199	204	209	215	220	225	230
5′ 1″	195	201	206	211	217	222	227	232	238
5′ 2″	202	207	213	218	224	229	235	240	246
5′ 3″	208	214	220	225	231	237	242	248	254
5′ 4″	215	221	227	232	238	244	250	256	262
5′ 5″	222	228	234	240	246	252	258	264	270
5′ 6″	229	235	241	247	253	260	266	272	278
5′ 7″	236	242	249	255	261	268	274	280	287
5′ 8″	243	249	256	262	269	276	282	289	295
5′ 9″	250	257	263	270	277	284	291	297	304
5′ 10″	257	264	271	278	285	292	299	306	313
5′ 11″	265	272	279	286	293	301	308	315	322
6′ 0″	272	279	287	294	302	309	316	324	331
6′ 1″	280	288	295	302	310	318	325	333	340
6′ 2″	287	295	303	311	319	326	334	342	350
6′ 3″	295	303	311	319	327	335	343	351	359
6′ 4″	304	312	320	328	336	344	353	361	369
6′ 5″	312	320	329	337	346	354	363	371	379
6′ 6″	320	329	337	346	355	363	372	381	389

Table 1.iii.: Body Mass Index Table for BMI 37-45

Normal Weight: BMI 18.5 to 24.9								
BMI	**46**	**47**	**48**	**49**	**50**	**51**	**52**	**53**	**54**
Height (In.)	Weight (lbs.)								
5' 0"	235	240	245	250	255	261	266	271	276
5' 1"	243	248	254	259	264	269	275	280	285
5' 2"	251	256	262	267	273	278	284	289	295
5' 3"	259	265	270	278	282	287	293	299	304
5' 4"	267	273	279	285	291	296	302	308	314
5' 5"	276	282	288	294	300	306	312	318	324
5' 6"	384	291	297	303	309	315	322	328	334
5' 7"	293	299	306	312	319	325	331	338	344
5' 8"	302	308	315	322	328	335	341	348	354
5' 9"	311	318	324	331	338	345	351	358	365
5' 10"	320	327	334	341	348	355	362	369	376
5' 11"	329	338	343	351	358	365	372	379	386
6' 0"	338	346	353	361	368	375	383	390	397
6' 1"	348	355	3633	371	378	386	393	401	408
6' 2"	358	365	373	381	389	396	404	412	420
6' 3"	367	375	383	391	399	407	415	423	431
6' 4"	377	385	394	402	410	418	426	435	443
6' 5"	388	396	405	413	422	430	438	447	455
6' 6"	398	407	415	424	433	441	450	459	467

Table 1.iv.: Body Mass Index Table for BMI 46-54

BMI is the most popular way to determine the amount of fat present in your body. Though it is not 100% accurate. For a bodybuilder, BMI may be an inaccurate representation due to increased muscle mass. However, BMI is considered "accurate enough" to get a quick snapshot of the fat tissue present. For most individuals, an increase in body weight typically means an increase in fat content. When losing weight, keep in mind that most of the weight loss is fat, some weight loss may also be muscle.

Now we have recognized how BMI is measured, let's look at the chart below to see what the BMI numbers actually mean.

BMI	Weight Class
Below 18.5	Underweight
18.5-24.9	Normal
25.0-29.9	Overweight
30.0 and up	Obese

Table 2: BMI and Weight Class

The higher the BMI, the more fat your body is storing. The healthiest BMI range for most individuals is between 18.5 and 24.9. An example would be if you were 5 foot 6 inches tall, your healthy weight range may be between 115 lbs. and 154 lbs. A person with the same height is considered overweight if they weigh in between 155 lbs. and 185 lbs. Being overweight puts you in a slight risk of weight-related diseases. Statistically, risk goes up significantly for the same person who is 5 foot 6 inches tall after 186 lbs.; where the BMI crosses the 30 mark.

An individual with a BMI of 30 or more is considered obese. Even with a BMI of 30, you are at a greater risk of diseases associated with obesity including a reduction in life expectancy. The greater the number, the higher the risks become. On average, the quality of life becomes lower with a higher BMI.

Let explore the benefits and disadvantages of using BMI.

Benefits of Using BMI

❖ Provides a quick and easy way to measure obesity.

❖ Help you use it as a compass to gauge your progress for your long-term weight loss goals.

❖ Helps determine the insurance eligibility for bariatric procedures.

❖ Factors in your height as it does not make sense to

use weight alone to track weight loss progress.

❖ It is a less invasive measurement when compared to other ways fat content is measured such as Dual Energy X-ray Absorptiometry (DEXA) and underwater weighing.

Disadvantages of Using BMI

❖ BMI may be an incorrect representation of fat content in bodybuilders and other athletes who put on more muscle mass than the average person. This is because the extra weight they put on is muscle mass and not fat tissue.

❖ Certain ethnic groups may have a lower BMI threshold. An example would be in the Asian population, it may be considered being obese at BMI of 27 instead of 30, when compared to the western populations.

❖ May not be an accurate representation of body fat in children in certain growth stages. Typically, doctors have charts that also factor in age to get a more accurate representation compared to using BMI alone.

❖ The measurement may not paint an accurate picture based on the distribution of fat. For example, a person whose body fat accumulation in the belly area is at higher risk for obesity-related illnesses when compared to the peripheral accumulation of fat (accumulation in the arms and legs).

Is It Easier to Put on the Extra Pounds Nowadays?

Now that we have covered the topic on what is obesity and how obesity is measured, let's explore what are the factors that are really making us fatter. We all know obesity is bad for our health. For some, it may just be embarrassing, for others, it may even be life threating depending on how severe the condition is. Losing weight may be summarized with a simple formula:

$$Eat\ Less + Exercise\ More$$
$$= Greater\ Weight\ Loss$$

Eating less and exercising more may be very easy to say but implementing this formula for weight loss may not be as simple. If it was this simple, then no one would be overweight.

So What Is Making Us Fatter?

The 8 enemies of weight loss:

1) **Accessibility of food** – Food is now available at more places than ever before. Fast-food restaurants are making meals fast and inexpensive. Processed food has a long shelf life and can be consumed at any time without any preparation. The microwave made it easy to heat up food making it very convenient to enjoy a late-night snack with no time-consuming preparation or cooking. Places that did not offer food before are now offering food. For example, during the great depression, theaters sold snacks to compete with other theaters to become more profitable. In fact, before that, popcorn was banned from movie theaters. Food availability is constantly increasing. It is now possible to order anything (and not just pizza anymore) online and have it delivered right to your door within minutes with popular ride sharing apps. Having a wider variety of food to choose from, it makes it harder for people to decide what food is healthy, especially that junk food is becoming a cheaper, easier, and a faster alternative to healthier options.

2) **Society has evolved on when and where food is consumed**. A few decades ago, a typical meal would be enjoyed with the family at the dinner

table. Nowadays, meals are readily enjoyed on the go, in front of the TV, and even while driving. One explanation may be that we have less time to enjoy the food since we are preoccupied with other factors that did not exist before. Smartphones, digital games, or the accessibility to thousands of tv shows and movies available on demand preoccupy much of our free time. With less free time and more choices available, it makes it harder and harder to set aside time to prepare and enjoy our food. This can increase mindless eating where we are not thinking about the food quality and quantity we are consuming. We may be distracted by watching a tv show or using our smartphones and not recognizing how much calories are actually being consumed making it easy to overeat and not even know it.

3)   **Lack of mobility** – Many jobs are becoming more and more stationary. We are just sitting too much! New and emerging technology is creating a more sedentary lifestyle as speed and ease of communication increases. Video chat, affordable transportation, remote controls, online shopping, and remote work only perpetuates the problem. In some industries, work from home is now possible where one can never leave the home and still live a normal life and make ends meet. Remember that our ancestors were hunters and gatherers were built for constant movement. No longer do we

have to exert the extra energy required for hunting or farming our food. This leads us to our next point, a lack of physical activity in our daily lives.

4) **Lack of physical activity** – Most of us don't get our daily exercise for one reason or another. Whether there are not enough hours in the day, lack of motivation, or other personal reasons, it is becoming increasingly difficult to get the recommended amount of physical activity.

5) **Increased portions** – More and more restaurants and food manufacturers are increasing the portions as a way to compete. The food industry is extremely competitive. One marketing trick they like to use is to increase the food portions as a way to build value for the consumer. This is especially visible in popular discount club stores where you can get everything cheaper if you buy in bulk. Restaurants are serving larger plates in response to competition as they don't want to look stingy as today's society is conditioned to think more is better.

6) **Ingredients that are not only addictive but also make you eat more** – Processed foods high in sugar, unhealthy fats, and refined grains make it much harder to lose weight. These types of foods

make it harder to satisfy hunger compared to healthier options that are high in fiber and protein. In fact, sugar can even change the brain chemistry to wire you to crave food even more. Therefore, cake and other sweets may become addictive as it makes us feel good. Sugar triggers our brain's reward system and can even create a dependence making us feel better[7]. Having a "sweet tooth" is just another way to say you have an addiction to sugar, making it much harder to lose weight.

7) **Drinks that contain sugar** – It is much easier to drink your calories than to eat them. Many fast-food places offer unlimited refills on soft drinks that further contributes to excessive calorie consumption. If we really think about it, when was the last time we satisfied our hunger with just liquid alone. It almost never happens. 48 oz. of a popular soft drink can contain as much as 556 calories. In fact, switching from soft drinks to zero-calorie drinks can have noticeable weight loss results in as little as one month. Try it!

8) **Other enablers** – Spouse, family members, and friends can be enablers to overeat. Many of us, when growing up, our parents told us to finish all the food on our plates as other parts of the world are not as fortunate. Leaving food on the plate has unconsciously become sort of taboo for many of

us. Other factors such as going out with friends can also contribute to over eating since we don't want to feel left out by being the only person not eating or drinking within the group. This makes it much harder especially when others don't understand your struggle with weight loss and may get the wrong message on why you are unable to join them. It is important to let others understand and communicate your weight loss goals so they can better under your situation and accommodate accordingly.

Obesity-Related Problems and Diseases

Now that we have explored some of the reasons which make us gain weight, let's explore the challenges and diseases obesity causes.

Reduced Life Expectancy

Did you know some life insurance companies have a weight chart that can put you in a more expensive premium tier? It's true, life insurance companies know the risk of dying is much higher in an obese individual versus someone is of healthy weight. For obese individuals, life expectancy is one of the consequences that they think about least. A 2016 Harvard University study revealed that individuals with a BMI between 35-40 had a 94% higher risk of mortality when compared to a someone with normal BMI. For those with BMI 40 or more, the mortality rate sharply rises. What was also interesting is that underweight individuals also had a higher risk of mortality[8]. The risk of premature death from obesity is similar to that of smoking. The lowest risk of death is within normal BMI limits (22.5 - 25). The reason for increased mortality is due to the combination of medical diseases that obesity causes, and other factors such as being more accident prone which we will discuss later in this chapter. It is important to note that BMI does not measure body fat, and that individuals who are athletes may have higher BMI but does not necessarily have an increased risk of death.

Medical Challenges

Obesity is known to cause or make worse a wide range of diseases. High blood pressure, heart disease, diabetes, stroke, sleep apnea, depression, abnormal levels of lipids in the blood, liver disease and even arthritis just to name a few. We will delve into some of the most common disease caused in-depth in the next chapter.

Disorders that are caused or made worse by obesity (but not limited to)
• Arthritis
• Asthma
• Blindness
• DVT (deep vein thrombosis)
• Depressions
• Diabetes
• Dyslipidemia
• GERD and Acid Reflux
• Gallstones
• Gout
• Hypertension
• Hypoventilation
• Infertility
• Intertrigo
• Ischemic Heart Disease
• Kidney Disease
• Lower back paint
• Non-alcoholic steatohepatitis
• Obstetric complications
• Peripheral neuropathy
• Polycystic ovarian syndrome
• Pulmonary hypertension
• Sleep apnea
• Some Cancers
• Stroke
• Urinary incontinence
• Venous ulcers

Table 3: Lists of Disorder That Are Caused or Made Worse by Obesity

Psychological Challenges

Obesity not only impacts our bodies negatively but also our minds as well. Many who are struggling with obesity may feel symptoms of depression, hopelessness, and even discomfort around others. Often when going out in public, the sense of other people looking or commenting at their weight takes a serious toll on mental health. This can lead to withdrawing from certain events, going out less in public, or even create isolation from the fear of being judged by others.

Isolation may help cope with the symptoms but deprives individuals from opportunities to go out with family, friends, and other social activities. It is common to find low levels of self-esteem in the morbidly obese individuals. Other challenges may include feelings of uselessness, worthlessness, disliking their appearance, and feeling unattractive to their partner or others.

Mobility and Physical Challenges

Performing common physical activities such as tying shoes or cutting toenails may be a very difficult or even an impossible task for the morbidly obese. Any sporting or physical activities can become very difficult. Tiredness, shortness of breath, and lack of flexibility make simple household tasks very challenging.

Being larger also limits the clothing they can buy off the rack, seating in public places (due to lack of bariatric furniture), and public transportation where you may require two seats or seatbelt extensions become necessary. Obesity can make ordinary tasks extremely difficult.

Economic Challenges

Studies show that people who are obese are at a higher risk of being accident prone, face higher rates of absenteeism in the workplace, and contribute to increased healthcare costs. Obesity is one of the largest contributors of rising healthcare costs in the United States. Current estimates show a range from $147 billion to $210 billion per year regarding the increased cost caused by obesity[9]. The increased risk of osteoarthritis, heart diseases and high blood pressure are the top contributors to the increased cost as these conditions are common in the morbidly obese population. Indirect factors, such as employment absenteeism, contributes to an estimated $4.3 billion[10] in additional cost not to mention lower productivity while on the job.

End of Chapter Worksheet

What is your current weight?

_____

What is your weight loss goal? The weight you would ideally like to achieve?

_____

_____

_____

_____

What is your current BMI?

_____

Name some of the reasons why you want to achieve your weight loss goal.

_____

_____

_____

_____

Name some of the personal secret reasons why you want to lose weight (things that you don't want others to know such as I want to be thinner and heathier than my friends).

_____

_____

_____

_____

Chapter 2. Obesity and The Benefits of Weight Loss

Weight loss is one of the most potent treatments in modern medicine. No other treatment compares when it comes to improving people's quality of life. It is one of the few treatments that actually reduces the chances of dying prematurely. The reason for this is that many diseases are caused or made worse by obesity. We have talked about the illnesses in the previous chapter that are associated with obesity, but let's dig a little deeper into the specifics and how weight loss can help improve or eliminate the associated illnesses.

Associated Illness Related to Obesity

Type 2 Diabetes

Type 2 diabetes is one the most common co-morbid conditions associated with obesity and is in the top ten leading causes of death in the United States. This lethal disease has been dubbed a silent killer since its symptoms are easy to miss. Ninety percent of individuals who have type 2 diabetes are overweight or have obesity. It commonly occurs in individuals who are gaining excessive weight or are obese where the excess calories are broken down into sugar. Excess sugar then goes into your blood, and your body needs to regulate the sugar levels to get them back to normal ranges. Your pancreas secretes insulin to keep your sugar levels in check, but after a while, your body cannot keep up with the insulin demand. Your body then develops a resistance to insulin which makes it very difficult to regulate the sugar levels and unable to do so efficiently anymore. Excessive glucose (high blood sugar) can cause your blood to stick in the blood vessels and damage other parts of your body.

Some of the most common complications associated with uncontrolled diabetes.

❖ Heart Diseases (Blood vessels that are damaged from excessive glucose can have adverse effects on your heart such as limited blood flow that can lead to a heart attack.)

❖ Blindness (blood vessels in the eye are damaged by the glucose. This can cause blurry vision and eventually lead to blindness)

❖ Infections

❖ Amputations (infections that have trouble healing. It can be severe enough that an amputation may be needed)

❖ Peripheral neuropathy (trouble getting blood to your legs where you may feel numbness or tingling)

❖ Kidney Disease

❖ High Cholesterol

Studies have shown that the higher the BMI, the higher the chance to have type 2 diabetes. It is common to see this disease resolve itself with weight loss, especially after bariatric surgery. Most treatments in modern medicine attempt to control the symptoms or limit the severity of illness. There is no treatment as powerful as weight loss for treating diabetes as it addresses the root cause.

Hypertension

Also known as high blood pressure, hypertension refers to the pressure blood applies to the inner walls of arteries. Blood pressure is typically measured as a fraction with two values, such as 140/100. The top number is the systolic pressure and the lower number is the diastolic pressure. The systolic pressure is measured when your heart is contracting to pump blood. Diastolic pressure (the lower number) measures the pressure when the heart is relaxing, and your blood is not as forcefully flowing.

The following table classifies the different categories for blood pressure:

Stage	Systolic		Diastolic
Normal	Less than 120	And	Less than 80
Prehypertension	120-139	Or	80-89
Stage 1 Hypertension	140-159	Or	90-99
Stage 2 Hypertension	160 or higher	Or	100 or higher
Hypertensive Crisis (Seek Emergency Care)	180 or higher	And/ Or	110 or higher

Table 4: Blood Pressure Range

Obesity is associated with hypertension and prehypertension. Hypertension is responsible for many other conditions that can adversely affect your life expectancy and overall quality of life. Medical treatment should be started if diagnosed with hypertension in order to minimize further complications. Weight loss has shown to lower blood pressure and can even decrease or even eliminate medication use. As you can see, weight loss can be one of the most powerful treatments in reducing high blood pressure and related diseases.

Dyslipidemia

Dyslipidemia refers to the abnormal cholesterol or fat (lipids) content in the blood. It is just a fancy term that describes elevated cholesterol/triglyceride levels that are outside the healthy range. The doctor may test these levels with a lipid panel (also known as a cholesterol test) to see if you are within healthy levels.

	Total Cholesterol	HDL Cholesterol	LDL Cholesterol
Good	170 or less	45 or higher	110 or less
Borderline	170 to 199	40 to 45	110 to 129
Higher	200 or more	---	130 or more

Table 5: Cholesterol Levels

Obesity increases the bad cholesterol (LDL) while decreases the good cholesterol (HDL) to abnormally low levels making it even harder for your heart to pump blood.

Acid Reflux / GERD

Acid reflux may be an important warning signal from your body of something that will get worse if ignored. Chronic acid reflux, sometimes referred to as GERD (Gastro Esophageal Reflux Disease) can lead to serious complications such as Barrett's esophagus or even esophageal cancer.

Common symptoms of acid reflux may include:

- ❖ Heartburn (may also be known as indigestion, a burning pain or discomfort that can move from the stomach all the way up to the chest or throat.)

- ❖ Regurgitation (The sensation of acid backing up into the mouth or throat. Also known as a wet burp)

- ❖ Bloating

- ❖ Nausea

- ❖ Dry cough

Studies have shown that obesity is an important risk factor in the development of gastroesophageal reflux disease (GERD). In some obese patients, the effects of

GERD can be so severe that drug therapy or surgery may be necessary to control the acid levels. Prolonged GERD can be deadly as it can lead to cancer if not treated in time. Many patients who have had the Lap-Band® procedure have reported immediate relief of GERD symptoms. The band placement is at the very top of the stomach, thus controlling the acid reflux. In fact, the Lap-Band® can be just as effective as other surgical treatments used to treat GERD making it an ideal choice for certain individuals who want to solve two problems with one procedure.

Sleep Apnea

Obstructive sleep apnea is common in the Western society. A recent National Health and Nutrition Examination Survey (NHANES) data document a dramatic rise in the prevalence of obesity, with prevalence estimates of approximately 60% (body mass index [BMI] > 25 kg/m3). More than half of individuals who suffer from sleep apnea are overweight or obese.

Sleep apnea, a common disorder associated with obesity, stops you from breathing for seconds to minutes during sleep. Typically, this episode of not breathing is stopped by coughing or snorting and can repeat itself up to 30 times per hour. The reduced oxygen intake and constant disruptions of sleep apnea can make it very difficult to get a good night's sleep. Individuals with sleep apnea commonly report lack of energy, focus and constant fatigue throughout the day. It also puts you at higher risk of having a stroke or heart attack. Weight gain has also been reported with sleep apnea which make things even worse.

The good news is that it is possible to treat sleep apnea with weight loss. Imagine not having to use a CPAP (continuous positive airway pressure) machine at night or waking up refreshed in the morning can be possible with weight loss.

Non-Alcoholic Steatohepatitis (NASH)

Non-Alcoholic Steatohepatitis is the inflammation of the liver that is associated with "fat" and not excessive alcohol consumption, commonly referred to with the acronym "NASH". NASH appears in obese individuals who have much of their weight distributed in their mid-section (apple-shaped body type). Not only is this disease commonly overlooked in the overweight / obese populations, it is also a leading cause for a liver transplant.

Psychological Disorders

According to the U.S. Centers for Disease Control (CDC), 1 in every 10 Americans deals with depression each year. Obesity can cause depression due to low self-esteem, social isolation and poor self-image. Obese individuals may feel helpless about their weight which can carry over to other aspects of life. Other symptoms may include being less outgoing, feeling tired, not caring about anything anymore, fear of being stereotyped, discriminated against or even ostracized. Others may see individuals struggling with obesity in a negative way whether intentionally or not. It can be very painful to deal with others who don't understand the struggle. Depression can even make obesity worse by triggering binge or emotional eating, especially when you are alone.

Infertility and Pregnancy

Obesity has been known to not only complicate pregnancies but also cause infertility in women, typically due to irregularities in ovulation. Polycystic Ovary Syndrome (PCOS) is also common in obese women where an increase in testosterone prompts excessive facial hair, acne, and period irregularities. Weight loss has been shown to help with these problems and can also help increase fertility.

Overall Quality of Life

As we have explored throughout this chapter, weight loss is a miracle treatment that can help eliminate or make certain obesity-related diseases more manageable. Measuring quality of life may be a difficult task, but hearing patient stories who have lost weight with surgical interventions such as the LAP-BAND® system, it becomes clear that their quality of life has significantly increased. They can now do the things that were very difficult or impossible before.

Here are some common things we hear from our bariatric patients that increased their quality of life:

❖ Ability to walk for longer distances
❖ No more chafing while walking
❖ Buying clothing at normal stores
❖ More outgoing and self-confidence
❖ No having to catch their breath from using the stairs
❖ Ability to tie their shoes
❖ Being able to cut their toenails without the help of someone else
❖ Not needing a seatbelt extension or special seating on an airplane.
❖ Having more energy
❖ Ability to play sports again
❖ Keeping up with people when they are walking
❖ Crossing your legs is now easy
❖ Sitting down on the floor to play with kids
❖ Getting more compliments
❖ Eliminate or reduced number of drugs needed every day
❖ Eliminate or reduced joint pain
❖ Ability to pick something up on the floor

Significant weight loss, as that achieved with the lap-band, can dramatically improve the quality of life for someone who is struggling with obesity.

Chapter 3. An Overview of Weight Loss Approaches

How We Lose Weight

There are essentially 2 ways that we can lose weight. We can decrease our calorie consumption, increase physical activity to burn calories, or do both. If you reduce the daily calorie intake to a number below our basal metabolic rate, weight loss will occur. Even though this sounds quite simple, it can be very difficult to achieve. Let's explore some options that can create this calorie deficit:

❖ **Diet** – diets can help you lose weight by reducing the amount of calories consumed.

❖ **Physical activity or exercise** – the more active you

are, the more calories you can burn.

❖ **Drugs** – Can help decrease your appetite, speed up your metabolism, or promote malabsorption helping reduce the overall calorie consumption.

❖ **Bariatric surgery** – or weight loss surgery is designed to help individuals lose weight when other options have failed. Bariatric surgery works by interfering on how your body absorbs calories (malabsorptive approach), physically restricts the amount of food that can be eaten in one sitting (restrictive approach) or both.

Now that we have outlined the four most common options that deal with weight loss, let's explore each one of them and weigh in the advantages and disadvantages of each.

Diets Don't Work (In The Long Run)

There are many diets that promise you to drop 15 pounds in a month or more. The reality is that fast weight loss is possible with dieting, but the results are usually temporary. When we lose weight fast, we are typically losing water weight. Therefore, it is so easy to put the pounds back on. In fact, research shows us that only 5% of individuals can successfully keep the weight off. Diets do work for short term, but for long-term, the odds are against you. There are many types of diets out there that help limit or shift the way we consume calories. Here are a few common diet approaches:

❖ **Low fat diet** – Fats have the most calorie content by weight, this diet type reduces the overall calories consumed.

❖ **Low-carb diet / high protein diet (Atkins)** – Carbohydrates are typically limited or removed from this diet to help reduce foods that contain high calories such as bread and pastas.

❖ **Low-sugar diet** – Reduces sugar consumption from empty calorie sources such as candy, desserts and other sweet snacks.

❖ **Low calorie diet** – Portion control of meals to limit the amount of daily calories consumed.

❖ **Meal replacements** (Example: Optifast®) – Helps limit the total calorie intake by replacing your meals with a shake or other low calorie, nutrient-rich medium.

❖ **Meal plans** (Example: Nutrisystem ®) – Just as other low-calorie diets, they promote easy portion control in order to limit the amount of calories consumed without the need to count calories.

Diets can potentially help people lose weight but are

typically temporary. How soon do you go from a specific diet to your normal eating habits? There are many reasons why this happens, you may get bored with a diet, always remain hungry or even unable to tolerate a diet long term (meal replacements are not a long-term solution). Others may feel deprived from the food they love such as bread, pasta, and sweets. Social situations are also major contributors to why diets are not followed. It is very hard to say no to a slice of cake at a birthday celebration of a loved one. For those reasons, diets are typically temporary unless they become part of your lifestyle.

Exercise Alone Is Not Enough

Even though exercise helps you stay healthy, keep your heart strong, and regulate your blood sugar, it is just not enough. For example, someone who is 250 lbs. and walks for 45 minutes at an average 3 mile per hour pace, will burn about 315 calories. A large 32oz soft drink has approximately 380 calories or a typical fast food burger at anywhere from 300 to 800 calories. Therefore, it is very difficult to burn off the excess calories while making bad food choices. Even if you can burn off the excess calories, it can be very difficult since there is just not enough time in the day to allocate toward exercise. For some who are struggling with obesity, exercise may be difficult, painful or embarrassing because they may feel others are watching. While others may find it very difficult to commit to a routine. After a month or two, they stop exercising altogether because results are not as expected especially due to poor diet choices.

Drug Therapy

They are many weight loss drugs out there on the market. Some are over the counter while others require a prescription. In today's society, it seems as almost anything can be solved with a couple of pills. But, when it comes to weight loss it is not that simple. A miracle drug has yet to be discovered that can completely treat obesity.

How Weight Loss Drugs Work

Weight loss drugs typically work by the following three mechanisms:

❖ **Malabsorption** – these types of drugs limit the amount of fat and nutrients that are absorbed when consuming food. They are designed to change your eating habits since eating certain food can cause severe diarrhea and other unpleasant side effects.

❖ **Boost metabolism** – work similar to a stimulant like caffeine where they increase your heart rate, pulse, and breathing. Side effects to these drugs may include insomnia and elevated blood pressure.

❖ **Appetite suppressants** – typically work by

increasing certain chemicals in our brain such as serotonin which can help with the feeling of fullness.

Drug therapy may not be right for everyone and there has not been enough studies to show significant long-term weight loss in morbidly obese individuals. Many of our patients have tried certain drug therapy before considering bariatric surgery. As with any drugs, some the side effects are not tolerable, or their weight loss results is just not enough. This makes it an impossible treatment option for many. Maybe someday we will have a miracle drug invented that will combat obesity more effectively. We can only hope.

Bariatric Surgery Options

Bariatric surgery is simply a fancy name for weight loss surgery. Let's explore exactly how bariatric surgery works. There are two main ways that bariatric surgery helps individuals lose weight.

Restrictive bariatric surgery, just as the name implies, restricts the size of your stomach. By limiting the amount of food you can eat at any one time, this will make you full faster. If you get full faster with less food, this will result in fewer calories consumed which will promote greater weight loss.

Examples of restrictive bariatric procedures include:

- ❖ LAP-BAND® System
- ❖ Gastric Sleeve
- ❖ Endoscopic Sleeve Gastroplasty
- ❖ Stomach Intestinal Pylorus Sparing Surgery (SIPS)
- ❖ Gastric Bypass (Rou-en-Y gastric bypass)
- ❖ Gastric Balloon
- ❖ Duodenal switch (DS) (also known as biliopancreatic diversion)

Malabsorptive bariatric surgery uses a different mechanism that limits the nutrient and fat absorption of food. This is typically done by rerouting the anatomy that allows the food to skip over certain areas where absorption happens which ultimately helps you lose weight.

Examples of malabsorptive procedures include:

- ❖ Gastric Bypass (Rou-en-Y gastric bypass)
- ❖ Stomach Intestinal Pylorus Sparing Surgery (SIPS)
- ❖ Duodenal switch (DS) (also known as biliopancreatic diversion)

Bariatric procedures can have multiple components (malabsorptive and restrictive) such as the gastric bypass, while others only have one weight loss mechanism such as the gastric sleeve (restrictive only). Now that we know the way bariatric surgery helps us lose weight, lets dive deeper and explore the risks and types of procedures available.

Types of Bariatric Techniques

When it comes to bariatric surgery, there are three types of surgical techniques. There is open surgery (traditional surgery), laparoscopic surgery, and endoscopic surgery.

❖ **Open surgery** – Before we had surgical cameras and fancy computer equipment, surgery was done by making cuts in to your abdomen to gain access to the components necessary for the bariatric procedure. The downside of open surgery is the increased risk of complications and can leave undesirable scars from the incisions.

❖ **Laparoscopic surgery** – This type of surgery involves making much smaller incisions in to the abdomen where the procedure is performed with the help of high definition cameras. This has been the choice for many surgeons as the smaller incisions lead to fewer complications compared to open surgery.

❖ **Endoscopic surgery** – although not a true surgical option, is the latest technique in bariatric procedures where a long flexible tube with a camera goes through the mouth down to the stomach with no abdominal incisions required. Procedures such as the Endoscopic Sleeve Gastroplasty and the gastric balloon utilize this new technique. Since this technique is less invasive then the other two, it has it benefits of faster healing and less downtime when compared to the other two options.

As with any surgery, bariatric surgery does carry risks. These risks include:

❖ **Death** – Death is always a risk when it comes to surgery. Bariatric surgery is considered safer than some other surgeries.

❖ **Embolism** – Blood clots can happen after surgery. This can lead to heart attack or stroke.

❖ **Infection** – infections resulting from incisions.

As with any choice in life, we have to weigh in the risks and the rewards. We also need to look at the risks of not having bariatric surgery to treat morbid obesity and associated conditions (diabetes, heart disease etc.) To many who are struggling with obesity, having bariatric surgery can help them achieve a better quality of life when other methods have failed.

Bariatric Procedure	Description
Vertical Sleeve Gastrectomy (Also known as the sleeve, gastric sleeve, or VSG)	This procedure is a relatively new with a moderate risk when compared to gastric banding and gastric bypass procedures. As a restrictive procedure, the sleeve gastrectomy limits the food intake by making the stomach smaller (in a shape of a "banana"). The excess portion of the stomach is then cut and removed. The gastric sleeve does not involve rerouting of the digestive tract.
Vertical Banded Gastroplasty (Stomach Stapling)	This procedure divides the stomach into two parts by using staples. The stomach pouch will be 10-15 percent of its original size. It restricts the amount of food intake.
Sleeve Plication	This procedure is similar to vertical sleeve gastrectomy, except the stomach is still intact and sewn shut, and not removed.

Bariatric Procedure	Description
Roux-en-Y Gastric Bypass (Also known as the gastric bypass, bypass surgery, and RYGB)	RYGB works by restricting food intake and by decreasing the absorption of food. Food intake is limited by a small pouch that is similar in size to the adjustable gastric band. In addition, absorption of food in the digestive tract is reduced by excluding most of the stomach, duodenum, and upper intestine from contact with food by routing food directly from the pouch into the small intestine.
Biliopancreatic Diversion With Duodenal Switch Gastric Bypass	Similar to the sleeve gastrectomy, this procedure begins with the surgeon removing a large part of the stomach. The valve that releases food to the small intestine is left, along with the first part of the small intestine, known as the duodenum. The surgeon then closes off the middle section of the intestine and attaches the last part directly to the duodenum. The separated section of the intestine isn't removed from the body. Instead, it's reattached to the end of the intestine, allowing bile and pancreatic digestive juices to flow into this part of the intestine.

Bariatric Procedure	Description
Adjustable Gastric Banding (Also known as lap-band, the LAP-BAND® System, gastric banding, or laparoscopic gastric banding)	In the laparoscopic adjustable gastric banding procedure, a band containing an inflatable balloon is placed around the upper part of the stomach and fixed in place. This creates a small stomach pouch above the band with a very narrow opening to the rest of the stomach, which is also known as the stoma. An access port is then placed under the skin of the abdomen. A tube connects the port to the band. By injecting or removing fluid through the port, the balloon can be inflated or deflated to adjust the size of the band. Gastric banding restricts the amount of food that your stomach can hold, so you feel full sooner, but it doesn't reduce the absorption of calories and nutrients.

Table 6: Quick Summary of Bariatric Procedures

Chapter 4. Lap-Band 101 – An In-depth Introduction

In chapter 3, we have talked about the different approaches to losing weight. In this chapter we will dive more in-depth into the LAP-BAND® system, discuss a brief history of gastric banding, and how gastric banding works.

The Evolution of the Lap-Band

One of the first gastric banding procedures was performed by Wilkinson and Peloso in 1978[12]. The procedure that they performed was non-adjustable and made from a 2cm Marlex mesh that was placed around the upper part of the stomach. In the 1980s, surgeons began experimenting with other materials including silicone. The challenge encountered during these early attempts at restriction showed a high failure rate due to lack of adjustability of the stoma, stomach slippage, food intolerance erosion, pouch dilatation, and intractable vomiting. Despite these complications, it was discovered that silicone was the best-tolerated material for gastric banding as it had far fewer adhesions and tissue reactions when compared to other materials.

About a decade later in 1986, Lubomyr Kuzmak, a Ukrainian surgeon was one of the first to report the clinical use of the "adjustable silicone gastric band" that was done via open surgery. Kuzmak, tried to solve the pitfalls of the previous gastric banding techniques by inventing a modified version of his original silicone non-adjustable band he had been using since 1983. By incorporating this adjustable feature to the band, clinical data showed improved weight loss and a reduction in complications when compared with the non-adjustable variants that he had used previously[13].

Later on, in 1991 Inamed with the help of talented bariatric surgeons, has focused on creating a safer and more effective laparoscopic version of the adjustable gastric band. Allergan bought over Inamed and took over the lap-band name. Once they have further improved the design, they began to teach other surgeons on how to perform this procedure in 1994 at the First international workshop on Laparoscopic Adjustable

Gastric Banding in Huy, Belgium. Further innovation by Allergan made it a popular choice by many surgeons worldwide. There have been a few iterations of the LAP-BAND® which further improved the safety and effectiveness. In 2013, Apollo Endosurgery acquired the Obesity Intervention Division from Allergan which included the LAP-BAND® device.

U.S. Availability and FDA Approval

Even though the LAP-BAND® has been available in other countries, it has not been until 2001 that the LAP-BAND® was approved by the FDA (Food and Drug Administration) as a treatment for obesity in individuals who have a BMI of 30 or higher. The FDA sets a strict standard before a specific treatment can be marketed. They review data to make sure that this treatment does what it says it does and also protect you from misleading marketing claims. As of 2018, the LAP-BAND® system from Apollo Endo is the only adjustable gastric banding product available in the United States.

Other Types of Lap-Band Products

In the U.S. market, there are two types of adjustable gastric bands have been approved by the FDA: LAP-BAND® and Realize™ Band. However, as of 2016, the LAP-BAND® is the only adjustable laparoscopic gastric band available in the United States. Realize™ Band, may also be known as the Swedish adjustable gastric band

(SAGB) by Johnson & Johnson, has been discontinued as of 2016[14].

Other alternatives such as the HELIOGAST® HAGA or the MIDBAND ™ are only available in Europe and are not approved the FDA.

The Differences Between the Lap-Band and the LAP-BAND®

Before going in any deeper, let's explore the differences between LAP-BAND®, and lap-band. The LAP-BAND® is a registered trademark of Apollo Endosurgery that refers to the branded version of a lap-band (short for laparoscopic adjustable band or any adjustable laparoscopic gastric band). We will be using the generic term of lap-band when discussing details about this tool to make it easier to understand. Occasionally, we will be using the branded term "LAP-BAND®" when we specifically are referring the Apollo Endosurgery's product.

How Does the Lap-Band System Work?

Now that we understand the evolution behind the lap-band system, let's explore how exactly it works. The lap-band is a restrictive procedure, which means that it limits the amount of food that you can eat at any one time making you feel full faster. This is done by placing an adjustable silicone ring around the top of your stomach, creating a smaller upper pouch known as the stoma. The stoma limits the amount of food that will go in to your main part of your stomach. The best part of the lap-band is that it is adjustable. Your surgeon can adjust the size of the silicon ring, tighter to restrict more food or loosen it up when needed.

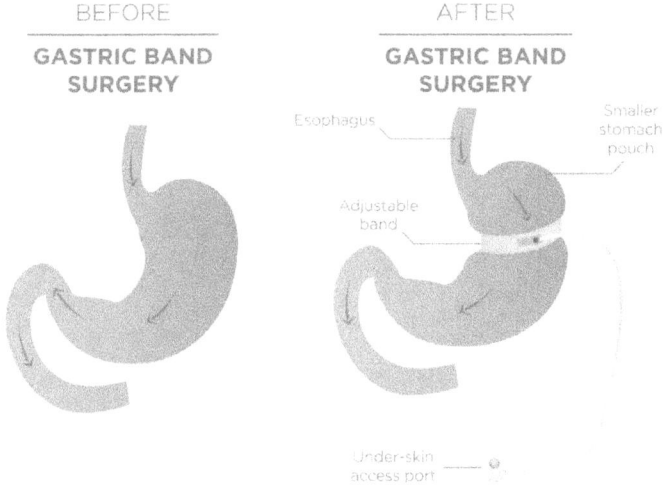

BEFORE

GASTRIC BAND
SURGERY

AFTER

GASTRIC BAND
SURGERY

Esophagus

Smaller
stomach
pouch

Adjustable
band

Under-skin
access port

Does the Lap-Band System Work?

In order to answer this question, we will need to first explore why humans get hungry. Humans have two type of eating drives, homeostatic and hedonic eating. Homeostatic eating is when our brain signals us to eat in order to stay alive. Food is converted in to energy to help our body function on a daily basis. These functions include pumping blood, repairing tissues, and even breathing. If we stop eating, we will eventually die.

Hedonic eating, on the other hand, is eating for pleasure. The enjoyment of food textures, flavors, and even social activities just to name a few. If we are sitting at a table full of yummy food, it is hard to stop ourselves from trying something, even if we just ate. This can also be described as non-hunger eating, which is a major contributor to excess calories that only worsen obesity. Our hypothalamus starts receiving inputs from various stimuli such as time of day (lunch time) seeing or smelling appetizing food or being invited to a social event where everyone is eating. Even though you may have just eaten, and not really hungry, these stimuli may lead you to feel hungrier and hungrier until you eventually give in.

Satiety vs. Satiation

Once we have just finished a meal, our brain gets signals that we are full, and not hungry anymore. This sense of not being hungry is defined as "Satiety". Satiation, on the other hand, is the feeling you get right after a meal that your hunger is under control. Even though the two words sound similar, it is important to note the difference to better understand how the lap-band works.

The lap-band creates a sensation of both satiation and

satiety. The band around the stomach creates a sense of satiety that is present throughout the day. It is common to hear my patients say that they do not feel hungry all the time anymore. The gastric band also creates satiation with smaller amount of food to trigger this response. This means that a smaller meal will satisfy the hunger where previously a bigger meal was necessary.

By controlling satiety and satiation effectively, less food will be consumed since you get full faster and stay full longer. In a way, think of the lap-band as rewiring your brain to eat less.

The Anatomy of the Lap-Band

Now that we have a basic understanding on how the lap-band works, let's explore the three main components of a modern lap-band system.

The Gastric Band

The gastric band is a circular ring that is made out of silicone. It is placed around the top portion of the stomach in order to make a stoma, the small upper pouch of the stomach. Saline is located in the inside of the gastric band which controls how tight the band is around the stomach. More saline will make the band snugger, while removing saline will loosen it up. Since everyone is different, this makes it perfect to adjust the band for a more custom fit.

Connection Tubbing

The connection tubing is a 50-centimeter (approximately 20 inch) tube made out of silicone. It acts as a conduit that carries the saline from the access port to the gastric band (or vice versa) that enables adjustment without surgery.

Access Port

The access port sits right below the skin and attached to the muscle of your abdomen. It allows the surgeon to insert a needle into the port to add or remove saline to make the necessary adjustment. Since this port is made out of silicone, it does not interfere with any imaging such as MRI or CT scans and won't set the alarm off during a TSA checkpoint. Some surgeons may use Fluoroscopy to find the port by using x-ray so that they can pinpoint the exact location of the port without the guesswork.

Chapter 5. Is The Lap-Band Right for You?

In this chapter, we will explore the benefits as well as the risks associated with the LAP-BAND® system including:

- The features and benefits of the LAP-BAND® system
- Lifestyle commitment component
- Risks vs. benefits
- Complications and side effects
- Can the lap-band fail?
- Eligibility and qualifications
- Contraindications
- Co-morbidities and the lap-band
- Lap-band vs other options

Remember that your doctor is the key component that can help you decide if the LAP-BAND® system is right for you.

Features and Benefits of the Lap-Band

The features that make the LAP-BAND® system a great alternative to traditional weight loss procedures and here is why:

The LAP-BAND® combats hunger in multiple ways

The primary way the lap-band works is by the restriction mechanism. The pressure created by the band on your stomach helps signal your brain that you are full. Your stomach capacity becomes reduced which will limit the amount of food that you can eat at any one time. The band will also make you feel full longer as you have the constant pressure applied to your stomach from the band. You will not feel as hungry between meals and smaller meals will be more satisfying.

What type of weight loss to expect with the LAP-BAND®?

On average, LAP-BAND® patients lose 65% of their excess weight at the 1-year mark[15] making it an effective way to lose weight gradually and keep it off long-term.

No Malabsorption

Procedures such as the Roux-en-Y gastric bypass take the malabsorptive approach where the nutrient absorptions from food is limited. This can cause severe side effects and may require a special vitamin therapy. The lap-band does not interfere with the nutrient absorption as the gastric bypass. This virtually eliminates the side effects of malabsorption.

Minimally Invasive

The lap-band is typically placed laparoscopically meaning that open surgery is not required unless complications occur. There is also no modification of the anatomy. Less scarring and faster healing are just some of the benefits compared to other more invasive bariatric procedures such as the gastric sleeve or the gastric bypass.

Adjustable

The key to the effectiveness of the lap-band is that it is fully adjustable. Adjusting the band can be done in minutes at the doctor's office without additional surgery. Adjustability is key to generate optimal results. The flexibility of tightening the band for further restriction or loosening the band for certain life events such as pregnancy where additional nutrition is required makes it an ideal choice for many individuals. Finding the best adjustment level enables us to achieve much better results while reducing unpleasant side effects.

Reversible

The lap-band procedure is fully reversible. We are not rerouting any of the body anatomies or removing any parts of the stomach as with other procedures, therefore we are not burning any bridges for future procedures. Although it is not recommended to remove the band as you may gain the weight back, the lap-band does give you the option to remove it if necessary.

Safer

The lap-band procedure is typically safer than other bariatric procedures (gastric sleeve, duodenal switch, gastric bypass) since no changes or body part removals are preformed such as cutting of the stomach or re-routing of the intestines.

Improve or Resolve Obesity-Related Diseases

The job of the lap-band is to help you lose weight more effectively than diet and exercise alone. Weight loss has been shown to treat or even eliminate certain obesity-related diseases such as type II diabetes.

Long Track Record

The FDA has approved the LAP-BAND® system since 2001 and is the only gastric banding system available in the United States as of 2018. Over 860,000 people worldwide have chosen the LAP-BAND® System to achieve lasting healthy weight loss, it is a solid option compared to other bariatric procedures in terms of safety and efficacy.

Lifestyle Commitment

It critical to understand that the LAP-BAND® system is only a tool and requires a lifestyle commitment to produce successful weight loss results. The LAP-BAND® is a very powerful tool that can help you lose the excess weight, but you will need to take responsibility and use it correctly. Think of getting the lap-band as a partnership with your surgeon and his or her medical staff. It is the surgeon's responsibility to place the band safely, accurately and securely. Your responsibilities include making healthy food choices, exercise regularly, do all the proper aftercare and follow-ups, stay in touch with your medical professionals, and have a strong support system to help you get the desired results. Everyone needs to do their part in order to achieve the best results. In Chapter 6, we will guide you on building out a team to make it easier for you to succeed.

Risks vs. Benefits

Now that we have identified the features and benefits of the lap-band, let's explore some of the risks associated. The lap-band is considered to be major surgery and is a life-changing experience. Even though the lap-band is a safer procedure other alternatives, serious risks and complications can occur. Therefore, is it important to learn about the possible risks before making a decision and have realistic expectations on the outcome. In this section, we will identify the risks related with getting the lap-band. To get the latest safety information, visit www.lapband.com

Risk of Death

As with any laparoscopic surgery, there is a risk of death. The risk of death with the lap-band is about 1 in 2,000 patients compared to 1 in 250 from the Roux-en-Y gastric bypass surgery. Certain factors such as age and other certain diseases may increase your risks. It is always best to let your surgeon know your full history to get a better idea of the risks associated. The most common reason for death due to bariatric surgery is from a heart attack after the procedure (due to blood clots).

If someone dies from a lap-band placement, it is due to a series of technical errors that would need to take place. To minimize the risk of death, select a surgeon who is extensively trained and has years of experience with a great track record. Request the surgeon's outcome data to help you better understand the risks. The lap-band is a safe procedure when done properly. Keep in mind that the potential risks can be higher when dealing with an inexperienced surgeon. Even though the data shows us the lap-band procedure is safer than other bariatric alternatives there is always a risk.

Complications Specific to the Lap-Band

Certain complications can occur with the lap-band, some more serious than others. Let's explore the most common type of lap-band related complications.

Slippage

The band can slide out or slip from the intended location. There are two ways the band can slip out of place. Anterior slippage is when the band slips in front of your stomach and posterior slippage which happens when the back of your stomach slides up through the band. When slippage occurs, stomach dilation happens which increases the size of the stoma. Food restriction is reduced rendering the lap-band ineffective. Individuals with a BMI of 40 or higher have a greater risk of slippage versus those with a lower BMI. Symptoms of slippage may include vomiting and acid reflux. If slippage occurs, it will be up to the surgeon to decide the course of action. Minor slippage can be corrected with deflation and re-inflation. It the slippage is serious; a reoperation may be necessary.

Erosion

Erosion occurs when the band works its way through the stomach wall. This happens when the band is not properly sitting in the groove that the surgeon makes during placement. If erosion takes place, the band will not be effective anymore. Typically, there is no acute illness of pain. Surgery will be needed to properly reposition the band to make it effective.

Leakage

Leakage occurs when the saline solution leaks out of the tubing or the access port. If leakage occurs, you will notice that there is little to no restriction. This can happen if the access port or tubing is damaged. Damage can happen if the needle punctures the port during the fill. It is important to note that you should NEVER fill the port yourself. Serious complications can occur. Always have a surgeon or a trained medical professional do the adjustment to minimize complications. Surgery is required to remove and replace the damaged tubing or port.

Esophageal Dilation

Esophageal dilation happens when the esophagus is overly stretched due to food regularly overflowing from the stoma and backing up to the esophagus. This may happen if you eat too fast or if the band is on too tight. It may feel as if you have a painful sensation behind your throat. The probability of this happening is higher with individuals with a higher BMI (>40). Esophageal dilation can be reduced by eating more slowly, chewing your food thoroughly, taking extra time in between bites, and being careful not to overeat. Esophageal dilation is treated by (partially or fully) deflating the band until the esophagus returns back to normal. Depending on the severity of the dilation, a reoperation may be needed to correct the dilation.

Gastrointestinal Symptoms

Gastrointestinal symptoms are common in lap-band patients. Here is a list of common symptoms that patients may experience:

o   Vomiting
o   Nausea
o   Dehydration (due to vomiting)
o   Diarrhea
o   Indigestion
o   Constipation
o   Abdominal pain
o   GERD / Acid reflux
o   Trouble Swallowing

Complications Table

The table on the next page provides a summary of common complications with the lap-band system. If you experience any side effects or symptoms, contact your surgeon immediately.

Problem / Complication	Estimated Occurrence
Death	~0.1%
Band Erosion	2.1% - 9.5%
Leakage	1.1% - 4.9%
Slippage	2% - 18%
Perforations	0.5% - 3.1%
Food Trapping	1% - 2%
Nausea and Vomiting	Up to 70%
Port Inversion / dislodgement	10.3%
Port Leak	1.1% - 4.9%
Port / Band Infection	1.5% - 5.3%
Port Dislocation	6.9%
Dilation	6.3% - 16.9%

Table 7: Lap-Band Problems and Complications.
Source: BariatricSource.com - https://www.bariatric-surgery-
source.com/lap-band-problems-lap-band-complications.html (October
2018)

Why the Lap-Band Can Fail?

Now that we have explored the complications and side
effects, let's see how and why the lap-band can fail. You
may have read online or have your friends or relatives

talk about how the lap-band does not work or that the lap-band is not effective anymore. You may have also been told by your doctor that the lap-band has been ineffective due to prior patient results. While failures can occur, as with any medical procedure, many failures can be easily avoided. But before we examine the reasons why the lap-band can fail, let define failure. There are three categories of failure: insufficient weight loss, lack of follow-up and removal of the band.

Insufficient Weight Loss

Insufficient weight loss can be defined as less than 25 percent of excess weight loss after 2-years of band placement. A thorough diagnosis is needed to see why the patient is not losing weight. It may be due to several factors such as a leak in the band, the band is not properly adjusted, not enough physical activity or exercise, wrong eating habits and food choices. We do not give up on these patients. Instead, we try to diagnose these patients to see what we can do to get them back on track.

Lack of Follow-Up

Follow-up is a critical component to effective weight loss. Patients who tend to skip follow-up are frequently associated with poor results. Proper follow-up is required to make sure you stay on track with your weight loss journey and to identify any complications before they may become more serious. Skipping follow-up also leads to improper band adjustments which can affect your weight loss results. Therefore, it is very important to regularly follow up with your surgeon (we recommend no longer than 6 months between follow-ups) for best results.'

Band Removal

Sometimes the lap-band needs to be removed due to complications such as band erosion. Other times, the patient chooses to have it removed since they feel as if the band is not working for them anymore. The great thing about the LAP-BAND® system is that it is fully reversible so that if in the future the patient would like to have the lap-band back again, this can be an option.

What Are the Requirements to Be Qualified for the LAP-BAND® System?

Not everyone qualifies for the LAP-BAND® system. You will need to meet certain eligibility criteria before you decide to proceed. Your doctor will need to need to be assured that you do not have any factors that can cause problems with the placement of the LAP-BAND® system.

BMI Requirement

You need to have a Body Mass Index (BMI) of at least 40 or have a BMI of 30 with one or more obesity-related comorbid conditions.

Age

You need to be at least 18 years old.

Weight Loss History

A history of prior unsuccessful weight loss attempts such as exercise, dieting, or drug therapy.

Other Conditions

You are currently not suffering from any other disease that may have caused your excess weight.

Alcohol / Drugs

You do not drink alcohol in excess and not addicted to drugs.

Mentally Prepared

You are prepared to make major changes in your eating habits and lifestyle.

Pregnancy

You are not currently pregnant (patients who become pregnant after their gastric band placement may require adjustments or removal).

Contradictions

Variety of factors may disqualify you from being a candidate for the LAP-BAND® system. It is always best to speak to a medical professional to review your qualifications. You may not be a good candidate if you have:

- ❖ Cirrhosis
- ❖ Chronic pancreatitis
- ❖ An addiction to drugs or alcohol
- ❖ An inflammatory disease or condition of the gastrointestinal tract (ulcers, severe esophagitis, Crohn's disease)
- ❖ Severe lung or heart disease
- ❖ Any disease that makes you a poor candidate for any surgery
- ❖ Problem that can cause bleeding in the stomach or esophagus. (dilated veins or telangiectasia)
- ❖ An Infection anywhere in your body.
- ❖ A history of chronic or long-term steroid use
- ❖ An allergy to the materials of the device
- ❖ An intolerance to an implanted device
- ❖ Portal hypertension

❖ An irregular / not normal esophagus, stomach or intestine. (example: narrow opening)
❖ Experienced an intraoperative gastric injury (example: gastric perforation at or near the placement location)
❖ An autoimmune connective tissue disease such as systemic lupus erythematosus or scleroderma. The same is true if you have symptoms of one of these diseases or if someone in your family has these types of diseases.

As you can see, the LAP-BAND® system is not for everyone. Check with your doctor if you have any of the following contradictions or other conditions that can impact your eligibility.

Co-Morbidities and Benefits of the Lap-Band

In previous chapters, we have discussed obesity-related diseases, and the associated health risks. The lap-band is a tool to help you lose weight which can potentially improve or resolve these co-morbidities. Let's revisit some of the obesity-related conditions the lap-band can help with:

❖ Type 2 Diabetes
❖ Hypertension (high blood pressure)
❖ Heart Disease

❖ Gastroesophageal Reflux Disease (GERD)
❖ Sleep Apnea
❖ Asthma
❖ Depression
❖ Overall Quality of Life

The LAP-BAND® system can be an effective tool to lose the excess weight to help improve or even eliminate the above disorders.

The Lap-Band vs. Other Options

Let's see how the lap-band stacks up against the four most common alternatives.

Lap-Band vs. Doing Nothing

If you do nothing about your weight condition, nothing will happen. The lap-band helps most people lose the extra weight.

Lap-Band vs. Diet and/or Exercise

Exercise or diet is only one piece of the puzzle and on their own are unlikely to help you lose weight and keep it off. Having a good diet and exercise plan is essential for long-term weight loss, but it is easier said than done. Diets can help you lose weight, but it may not be a long-term solution. The lap-band is a tool that helps you limit your food intake and makes you feel full faster and stay full longer. It works together with healthy food choices and exercise to help boost weight loss results.

Lap-Band vs. Medication

The problem with medication is that it is temporary and not a long-term solution. Many weight loss medications can only be taken for no more than 12 weeks at a time. They also can have unwanted side effects which may not be an option for some.

Lap-Band vs. Other Bariatric Procedures

When comparing the lap-band to other traditional bariatric procedures such as the gastric sleeve or the gastric bypass the lap-band has unique benefits. These benefits include:

❖ **Adjustability** – the band can be adjusted to fit your weight loss goal.

❖ **Reversibility** – no bridges are being burnt, even though the lap-band is designed to be permanent, it can be removed if necessary.

❖ **Does not alter anatomy** – other bariatric procedures alter your body's anatomy which can cause more complication.

Now that we have explored the benefits and risks of the

LAP-BAND® system, this information should be helpful in deciding if the lap-band is a good fit for you. In the previous chapters we have explained how losing weight can help improve your overall quality of life, improve or eliminate obesity-related co-morbidities, and help increase your life expectancy. We have also gone over the qualification for eligibility of the LAP-BAND® system and the contradictions to see if you are a good fit. In the next chapter, we will talk about how to build a team that enables you to succeed with your lap-band journey.

Chapter 6. The First Steps: Preparing for Bariatric Surgery

Chapter 6 will guide you step by step on how to prepare for bariatric surgery. As you will see, it will be structured a bit different than the other chapters as t first step for preparation is building out a team that will help you with your weight loss journey. This team will consist of the following:

❖ Your loved ones (family)
❖ Friends and colleagues
❖ Bariatric practice and medical professionals (surgeons, nurses, bariatric coordinator, dietitians, and others)

Choosing the right people will help you make a better-informed decision and support you through your weight loss journey. There are questions after each section to help guide you.

Team 1: Your Loved Ones

Your loved ones such as your spouse, kids, and other family members may be worried if you decide to have weight loss surgery. Certain changes after the surgery may be difficult to adapt to at first. Such changes may include alternative eating habits that can affect everyone in the family. Keeping them informed and including your loved ones every step of the way will help out a lot in your journey. Bring them to your appointments, informational sessions, and support group meetings. When everyone is on the same page, it will make your weight loss journey much easier.

List your family members that are closest to you and list how they will be an important part of your weight loss journey.

_____

_____

_____

_____

_____

_____

_____

Will they support you if you decide to have weight loss surgery? If not, why not?

_____

_____

_____

Will there be anyone who can make it difficult for you? If so, why?

_____

_____

_____

What do you think you will need from them in order for you to succeed in your weight loss journey?

_____

_____

_____

_____

Team 2: Your Friends and Colleagues

Your friend and colleagues are also an integral part of your journey. Everyone has their own opinion on weight loss surgery, therefore it is important to think about who you are going to tell.

How will sharing your weight loss journey affect your friendships?

_____

_____

_____

Who do you trust to share your weight loss surgery journey with?

_____

_____

_____

_____

Which one of your friends will be there to support you?

_____

_____

_____

_____

_____

Who do you think will make it difficult in your journey?

_____

_____

_____

_____

Who would you regret telling?

_____

_____

_____

_____

_____

Team 3: Bariatric Practice and Medical Professionals

Selecting the right bariatric team is critical for your weight loss success. If you have HMO, you will typically need a referral from your primary care physician, also known as the PCP. Your PCP may recommend a weight loss surgery specialist or other alternatives.

Is your doctor supportive of weight loss surgery?

_____

_____

What is your doctor's view on the lap-band procedure? Does he or she have any patients that have had the lap-band procedure done? If so, how was the outcome?

_____

_____

_____

_____

Did your primary care physician recommend a weight loss surgeon? If so, does the surgeon have good experience with the lap-band procedure?

_____

_____

_____

Is the recommend weight loss surgeon board certified? Affiliated with the (Metabolic and Bariatric Surgery Accreditation and Quality Improvement Program (MBSAQIP)?

_____

_____

How accessible is the surgeon? How about their staff? Is it easy to get an appointment?

_____

_____

What was your first impression of during your first visit with the surgeon? Did you feel safe and comfortable? Were all your questions answered?

_____

_____

_____

_____

Are there other bariatric surgeons in the practice? If so, which surgeon would perform your surgery? What are their credentials and experience?

_____

_____

_____

_____

_____

How will the aftercare be handled? Where will the aftercare take place? (examples of aftercare may include: adjustments, support group meetings, nutritional and psychological counseling)

_____

_____

_____

Are there other patients you can talk to who had the lap-band procedure? What questions would you like to ask them?

_____

_____

_____

_____

_____

_____

Is the recommended surgeon covered by your insurance? Do you have bariatric coverage? What would be your out of pocket expenses?

_____

_____

_____

How are the online reviews of the bariatric surgeon and the bariatric practice? You can typically Google the surgeon's name or the practice with the word "reviews" after their name to see the latest reviews. List each source and the rating. (example source: Healthgrades, Yelp, Google Reviews, Facebook etc.)

_____

_____

_____

_____

_____

Attending your informational seminar

When and where is the next bariatric informational seminar?

_____

_____

_____

_____

Who will you bring with you to this meeting and why?

_____

_____

_____

_____

_____

List the questions that you will ask at the informational seminar:

_____

_____

_____

_____

_____

What did you learn during the informational seminar that you did not know about before?

_____

_____

_____

_____

Which staff members did you meet at the Informational seminar? What did you think of them? Did they answer all the questions that you had?

_____

_____

_____

_____

_____

Chapter 7. What to Expect Before Lap-band Procedure?

Now that you have taken your first steps in getting a referral from your primary care physician (if necessary), building out your support team and attending a bariatric informational session. The next step is to schedule your pre-op appointment with the surgeon.

Your Pre-Op Appointment with the Bariatric Surgeon

During your pre-op appointment with the surgeon, it is important to establish a great relationship and trust.

Remember that your life will be in his or her hands. It is best to write everything down you would like to ask the surgeon on a sheet of paper so you would not forget anything due to being nervous or excited. Don't be afraid to ask the important "what if / hypothetical" questions such as "what if I go out of the country on vacation", the more you know about the procedure, the better.

Your medical history will be reviewed during your appointment, such as any test results, medical treatments, and previous surgeries. Always be transparent with your surgeon about any other treatments you may have had in the past, any medications you are taking both prescription and over the counter including any supplements or vitamins that may sometimes not show up on the medical records. It is critical the surgeon knows your full medical history to see if you are a candidate for lap-band surgery and if any previous conditions that can interfere. Just because you may have something that stands out does not automatically disqualify you from a bariatric procedure. Here are some things that often get overlooked and are important for your surgeon know before the procedure:

❖ Over-the-counter medications (including any pain relievers such as Motrin or Tylenol) and prescription medications. Since you will not be able to eat solid foods right after surgery, some medication may need to be crushed or taken in other forms such as a gel or powdered form. Always ask your medical professional as some medications may have special requirements and cannot be simply crushed.

❖ Supplements, vitamins, minerals, health powders, any kind of nutritional smoothies or anything that you would find at a health supplement store.

❖ Any oral contraceptives – alternative methods may be necessary.

Insurance

Have a clear communication channel with your health insurance provider to understand what procedures, tests, and assessments are covered and what is out of pocket to minimize any surprises. Every insurance plan and provider is different and may have special coverage and requirements. Some insurance providers may require you to take extra steps before approving your procedure. Make sure to not only know the total out-of-pocket costs, but also the requirements necessary for maximum reimbursement.

Medical Tests

There is a wide range of medical tests your doctor may order in order to approve you for a surgery. Here is a list of some of the test they may be done. The type of medical tests performed will be up to your doctor and surgeon to decide.

- ❖ Chest X-ray / Chest CAT scan
- ❖ Gastrointestinal (GI) X-Rays
- ❖ Gallbladder ultrasound
- ❖ Electrocardiogram (EKG)
- ❖ Blood sugar tests
- ❖ Liver function test
- ❖ Calcium test
- ❖ Carbon dioxide test
- ❖ Nutrient blood test (Key nutrients such as B-12, folic acid, Vitamin D.)
- ❖ Electrolyte blood test
- ❖ Kidney tests / BUN test

Psychological Assessments

Psychological assessments are done to evaluate your mental preparedness of the lap-band procedure as well as your mental stability. Untreated psychological disorders, such as untreated depression, may make it more difficult after the procedure. Losing weight or dealing with new challenges you may encounter may become harder to deal with. Don't think of psychological exams as something scary, or that you are a crazy person, they are there to identify any issues that may become unnecessary challenges later on. Be sure to answer all questions truthfully and to the best of your ability. Don't withhold any information as this will only hurt yourself. There are no right or wrong answers.

Meetings with Your Dietician

Your first appointment with the dietician will typically involve a dietary assessment on your current eating habits. The job of the dietician is not to point fingers but to better understand your diet situation and help you succeed by making suggestions on how to improve your diet and lower your overall calorie intake.

Some of the talking points may include:

- Portions / Serving sizes
- Current and past eating habits
- Eating out habits (going to restaurants)
- Understanding nutritional labeling
- Being conscious of everything that you eat
- Understanding calorie intake
- Dietary supplements
- Keeping a food log

After better understanding your dietary habits, your dietitian will talk about the pre-op and post-op diet to get you better prepared and let you know what to expect.

The Pre-Op Diet

Your surgeon may request you to lose weight or not to gain additional weight before the surgical placement of the gastric band. Losing weight before surgery can reduce the size of an enlarged liver back to its normal size which can make the surgery safer. An enlarged liver can make it difficult to place and position the lap-band around your stomach. The pre-op diet is designed to prepare you for surgery. It is typically required by your surgeon or insurance company as it shows that you are committed to making a lifestyle change and provides proof that you can follow a low-calorie diet. Most importantly, it will help you transition to your post-op diet.

The pre-op diet typically consists of 800 – 1200 calories per day plan that you will have to do for a few weeks to a couple of months. Once you get closer to your surgery date, you may be required to go on a liquid diet depending on your dietician or surgeon's requirement. Every surgeon and dietician are different in terms of what you can and cannot eat, so make sure to follow your surgeon's and dietician's orders.

Start an Exercise Routine

Starting an exercise routine a few months before surgery may help you burn more calories and lose extra weight. It can make you feel healthier and help you feel stronger. You don't have to go on a crazy exercise routine, it can be something light like walking, performing chores around the house, gardening, etc. As with any new exercise routine, contact your doctor for approval. Adding physical activity to a healthy diet can help you lose more weight.

What to Expect During the Surgery

At this point, you have prepared and have scheduled your lap band procedure, we will discuss what will go on during the procedure. The surgery typically takes less than an hour and will be done under general anesthesia.

The lap-band is almost always performed laparoscopically but in rare occasions, it can be converted to an open surgery if complications occur or if there are too many adhesions from previous surgical procedures. During open surgery, the placement of the lap-band will be done virtually the same but generally patients may experience more discomfort when compared to laparoscopic placement. A longer hospital stay is to be expected if done via open surgery.

How Is the Procedure Performed?

The LAP-BAND® system, being a laparoscopic procedure, means that only tiny incisions are made in the abdomen to perform the surgery. These tiny incisions are typically 0.2 in (5mm) across so that the surgeon can place the camera and instruments in order to perform the procedure. Since the incisions are so small, when they heal, they are almost invisible.

Now with the camera placed inside your abdomen, the surgeon can then see everything inside required to perform the procedure making it much less invasive than traditional open surgery. The surgeon will then place an adjustable gastric band around the upper portion of your stomach. A small pouch is created, also known as the stoma, that limits the amount of food you can eat at any one time.

The access port, a critical component of the lap-band that allows easy adjustment, is placed inside the abdominal wall. To place the access port, the surgeon typically creates a larger incision in the skin of around one and a half inches wide. The location of the port is slightly left of the center belt line making it easier for the surgeon or medical professional to find during an adjustment. Being a larger incision, this area may be a bit tender after the procedure.

Post-Surgery

Once you wake up from the operation, you may feel discomfort. One location of discomfort commonly reported is in the stomach area due to the incisions, especially around the access port. Other commonly reported pain is the left shoulder. Even though we don't know exactly why there is pain coming from this area, we do know that it actually originates from the diaphragm. This type of pain is known as referred pain as brain thinks that the pain originates from a different area of the body than it actually is. You may be given a pain reliever or hot packs to help ease the discomfort.

After waking up, you may notice an intravenous (IV) drip to help keep you hydrated. Once you start drinking fluids such as water or tea without too much difficulty, we will then remove the IV. Generally, you will get out of bed and go for a quick walk shortly after the procedure as early mobilization is likely to have a smoother recovery.

A barium swallow, which is an X-ray examination, may be done to check if the band is in the correct position. Depending on the surgeon, it may or may not be performed, but it provides a way to diagnose any problems with the operation early on.

You may go home in as little as 2-3 hours, sometimes an overnight stay may be recommended. Before going home, you may be instructed on the new rules of eating with the lap-band, especially for the next few weeks when you will be transitioning from a liquid to a solid food diet. It is important to follow the lap-band diet to minimize any complications that can occur. Once home, you should be able to return to normal activities within 1-2 weeks.

Chapter 8. The Lap-Band Diet (Post-Op)

Diet Plan After the Lap-Band Surgery

The following dietary guidelines are designed for bariatric patients who are preparing after the Lap-Band procedure. Following these guidelines may help reduce complications, maximize the weight loss results, and boost your weight loss goals. As with any diet plan, consult with your doctor and dietitian before implementing this or any other diet plan.

The first few weeks after surgery, you may experience

mood changes and frequent irritability. However, it is crucial to follow your surgeon's instructions to reduce the post-operative complications such as nausea, diarrhea, dehydration, constipation, and band erosion. Schedule a post-operative consultation with your doctor and seek approval before progressing to the next diet stage.

Clear Liquid Diet

First Week After Surgery

For the first week after surgery, you are allowed only to consume clear liquids. You need to stay hydrated. Try to aim for 64 oz. of fluids daily. However, for the first couple days, you may progress from 24 oz. of fluids daily to 64 oz. to help your body adjust. Sip slowly, and you should stop drinking when you feel full.

EXAMPLES OF A CLEAR LIQUID

- Drinking water and no-calorie flavored water
- Ice chips
- Sugar-free popsicles
- Crystal light
- Sugar-free Kool-Aid
- Diet Snapple
- Clear protein drinks

Full Liquid Diet

Weeks 2-6 after surgery

Continue drinking fluids from the clear liquid diet. However, in this stage, you can add more liquid varieties to your daily intake. Keep in mind that your body still needs to heal, thus only liquids are allowed and non-chunky/particles foods.

❖ Drink slowly, take a few sips, and do not use a straw
❖ Stay hydrated. Try to drink at least 8 cups (64 oz.) of liquids daily
❖ Do not force yourself to drink when you feel full
❖ Take vitamin supplements as instructed by your doctor or dietitian
❖ Avoid sugary, alcoholic, and carbonated drinks

EXAMPLES OF A FULL LIQUID

- Everything from the clear liquid list
- Decaf tea and coffee
- No sugar added juices such as apple and carrot juice
- Sugar-free popsicles
- Sugar-free gelatin
- Low-calorie protein shakes
- Tomato puree soup
- Sugar-free pudding
- Nonfat milk and nonfat lactose-free milk

- Nonfat yogurt
- Applesauce, smooth variety without the chunks

Solid Foods

Week 7+

Week seven and beyond, after the placement of the lap band, involves the transition from full liquid to solid foods. Chew thoroughly and swallow your food slowly. Now you can introduce new healthy solid foods, one at a time.

❖ Include lean protein in your meal. Protein helps your body to maintain muscle mass, prevent hair loss, and provide energy. Some of the examples are chicken breast, turkey breast, fish, and soy products.

❖ Do not overeat. Cut your food into small pieces and chew thoroughly. Wait 10 minutes and see if you are full. When you feel full, you should stop eating. Stop eating when you are a 5 on the hunger scale (Table 8 – located later in this chapter).

❖ Eat three meals daily.

❖ Avoid drinking water for at least 30 minutes before and after a meal.

❖ Avoid fried foods, sugary desserts, crackers, sodas, and alcoholic beverages.

❖ Stay away from heavy cream. If your recipe requires heavy cream, substitute with nonfat or low-fat version.

❖ Choose low-fat cheeses over regular or whole milk cheeses.

❖ Take daily multivitamins as directed by your physician.

❖ Plan on what you eat before going out.

❖ Track your daily intake by having a food log/diary.

❖ You can eat bread, rice, pasta, non-crunchy cereals, soft crackers in moderation.

❖ Choose easy to digest vegetables such as cooked beets, green beans, mushrooms, zucchinis, and eggplants.

EXAMPLES OF SOLID FOOD

- Fresh apple slices
- Fresh cucumber slices
- Lean beef steak
- Grilled chicken breast
- Grilled fish
- Steamed fish
- Cooked spinach
- Cooked carrots
- Chopped Salad
- Mini turkey meatballs
- Soft or hard-boiled egg

*Nothing crunchy, crumbly, slimy or slippery such as macaroni & cheese, chips, pretzels, popcorns, trail mix, granola bars, lean cuisine, cereal, crackers, cream of wheat, oat meal, grits, and nutritional bars.

Dietary Plan After Lap-Band Adjustments

After each band adjustment, you need to go back to a liquid diet for about three days, then progressing to solid foods. Contact your doctor if you experience vomiting after a meal. Follow up with your doctor regularly.

THE HUNGER SCALE
1. Your stomach acid is churning, and you feel very weak.
2. You feel uncomfortable and irritable.
3. Your stomach is growling and you are hungry.
4. You feel a little hungry and uncomfortable.
5. Satisfied and comfortable, but you could eat a little more.
6. Satisfied and comfortable.
7. Full.
8. Bloated and full.
9. Uncomfortably full.
10. Stuffed. You are so full, you feel sick.

Table 8: The Hunger Scale

How We Should Eat

Ways to prolong meals and reduce the amount of food eaten.

- ✓ Eat slowly and savor each mouthful – take a small bite and chew it very well. Large chunks or not fully chewed food could stretch the area above the band. Develop a habit to enjoy the food and savor ever bite.

- ✓ Put down the fork between bites

- ✓ Delay eating for two to three minutes and converse with others

- ✓ Postpone a desired snack for 10 minutes

- ✓ Serve food on a smaller plate – a smaller plate will not allow you to pile on food reducing the guilty feeling of leaving too much food on the plate.

- ✓ Leave one or two bites of food on the plate – once you feel satisfied stop eating.

- ✓ Eat 2 to 3 meals per day. No snacking.

- ✓ Take 1-2 bites, wait 10 minutes before you take your next bite.

✓ Choose bulky food that will leave you full and satisfied longer.

✓ DO NOT drink your calories: Only water, crystal light, or sugar-free drinks. Stay away from soda.

✓ Wait 45 minutes after you take the last bite of your meal before you drink any liquids.

Coping with Food Triggers

- Eat only sitting down at one designated place
- Sit in a different seat at the table
- Leave the table as soon as eating is done
- Do not combine eating with other activities, such as reading or watching TV
- Do not put bowls of food on the table
- Do not keep trigger foods at home
- Keep all food in cupboards where it cannot be seen
- Shop for groceries from a list after a full meal
- Limit the amount of money taken when shopping
- Plan meals and snacks
- Plan for special events, parties, and dinners
- Freeze leftovers in individual containers
- Ask others to monitor eating patterns and

provide positive feedback
- Substitute other activities besides snacking

Bariatric Recipe Modification List

Ingredient	Substitution
1 cup whole milk	1 cup skim milk
1 cup evaporated milk	• 1 cup evaporated skim milk or • 1 cup skim milk + 1 cup nonfat dry milk powder
1 cup buttermilk	1 cup lukewarm skim milk + 1 tablespoon juice or vinegar. Let stand for 5 minutes, beat briskly
1 cup cream or half & half	1 cup evaporated skim milk
1 cup sour cream	• 1 cup nonfat sour cream or • 1 cup nonfat plain yogurt or • 1 cup 1% cottage cheese whirled in blender with 1 tablespoon of lemon juice
1 cup cream cheese	• 1 cup nonfat cream cheese or1 cup light pot cheese or • 1 cup whipped 1% cottage cheese

Ingredient	Substitution
1 whole egg	• 2 egg whites or • ¼ cup egg substitute
1 oz. unsweetened baking chocolate	3 tablespoons cocoa powder + 2 teaspoons vegetable oil
1 cup whole milk ricotta cheese	• 1 cup part-skim ricotta cheese or • 1 cup 1% cottage cheese
Mayonnaise	• Nonfat mayonnaise or • Nonfat plain yogurt
1 tablespoon butter or margarine	2 teaspoons canola oil
1 cup solid shortening	2/3 cup liquid canola oil
1 cup margarine	¾ cup canola oil
Oil for sautéing	• Nonstick spray or • Bouillon, wine, or water
Oil in salad dressing	Vinegar, nonfat yogurt, buttermilk, lemon juice, tomato juice
Nuts (in gelatin salad)	Chopped celery, carrots, or water chestnuts
Sugar	No calorie sweeteners
Fat	Try replacing fat with an equal amount of light or dark corn syrup, honey, pureed fruit (i.e. banana, thick applesauce, prunes)

Table 9: Bariatric Modification List

Chapter 9. Exercise

As discussed earlier, weight loss depends on the amount of food you eat (calorie intake) and the amount you exercise (calorie expenditure). You lose weight when your calorie intake is lower than your calorie expenditure. Therefore, combining exercise with healthy eating habits will boost your weight loss efforts. Exercise is a vital component to any successful weight loss program. However, that doesn't mean that you need to start training for a marathon on your way home from surgery. Start slow, take baby steps, and work your way up to at least 30 minutes of exercise a day. We want you to make a commitment and set this time aside every day for exercise unless restricted by a health problem.

You don't have to run or do intensive workouts for 30

minutes a day, it can be something as simple as a gentle walk on the treadmill. Start with low impact physical activity. The key is to get your heart pumping and adapt to a more active lifestyle. Try out different forms of exercise to see what works best for you. Create an exercise log to track your physical activity. If you miss any days, make up for them. Don't make up excuses on why you did not exercise. Daily exercise can help:

- Boost your metabolism
- Increase or maintain your weight loss
- Increases your energy
- Helps lower blood pressure
- Reduce your risk of developing heart disease
- Promote joint stability and bone strength
- Develop endurance, muscle tone and strength
- Make daily tasks easier (such as climbing stairs)
- Elevate your mood and even reduces stress
- Improve your overall health and quality of life

Here are a few strategies that that can help you stay interested in your workout:

❖ **Start slow** and continually increase your workout time or intensity (without putting yourself at risk of injury)

❖ **Adjust exercises** that make it more enjoyable for you. If you prefer walking to swimming, feel free to do more walking. Just keep in mind that some exercises help you burn more calories than others.

❖ **Keep the workouts simple**. You don't have to go and buy expensive gym equipment or hire a personal trainer. If you can afford a personal trainer it would be great but don't use that as an excuse to not exercise.

❖ **Listen to your favorite music** or audio books while working out. It can make your workout more interesting.

❖ If you are comfortable, **get your friends involved** with exercise. You can go to the gym together or join them on a morning jog.

❖ Work your way up to **at least 30 minutes of exercise** per day. Ideally you would want to have go up to 1 hour every day as long as you feel comfortable with that.

❖ You don't have to do the full 30 minutes at a time. **Feel free to split up your work out** in 10 minute increments throughout the day if that work better.

❖ **Most Important – No Excuses!** Create a routine and stick with a routine. If you miss any days, make up for them the following day. No doing your daily exercise because you were sick, on vacation, or did not have time are not valid excuses.

Remember that the lap-band is only a tool that helps you lose the weight by limiting how much food you can eat at any one time. The lap-band by itself will not make you lose weight, but when combined with the proper diet and exercise, it can help you lose weight faster and more effectively.

Here are more ideas to help you increase your physical activity

❖ Use stairs instead of taking elevators or escalators.
❖ Park your car farther from your intended destination.
❖ If you can, see if you can use alternate methods of transportation. Chose walking or biking over driving when possible.
❖ Go on a nature tour at a local park or forest preserve. Explore your local city by walking or bike riding.
❖ Water aerobics and swimming provide great exercise with low impact on the body and joints.
❖ Housework or outdoor activities such as gardening are great opportunities to be active.
❖ Find an active hobby. Move away from sedentary activities such as watching TV or using a computer.
❖ Sports can be fun and help you stay fit.
❖ Join a local gym and exercise with like-minded individuals.
❖ Try Yoga. It is low impact and has many positive

benefits including building muscles and reducing stress.

Be creative in finding ways to be active. What activities do you enjoy?

_____

_____

_____

_____

_____

_____

_____

_____

Monthly Exercise Log

	Week 1	Week 2	Week 3	Week 4
Sunday				
Monday				
Tuesday				
Wednesday				
Thursday				
Friday				
Saturday				

Chapter 10. Living with The Lap-Band

Living with the lap-band can be very rewarding as this tool helps you lose more weight when used properly. One of the unique features to the lap-band is the adjustability aspect. Proper adjustments are key to maintain proper weight loss with the lap-band. There will be at times that you will need to increase the fluid in the band (making it tighter) when you start gaining weight again or notice that you are eating too much. Reducing the fluid volume is also be an option if you need additional nutrition for when you are pregnant, or if the band is too tight causing difficulty swallowing. Having proper follow-up is essential with the lap-band so that the surgeon can adjust the band to the optimal level for best results.

Your First Adjustment

Your first adjustment is typically performed 4 weeks after band placement. When the band is first placed, it is initially filled with approximately 3ml of saline, this is known as the basal amount. The exact amount to be filled will be determined by the surgeon, which may be more or less fluid. The basal amount of fluid is designed to help the band settle into the proper position during the initial placement. During the first week, you may have almost no desire to eat. This is where you may lose the most weight in a fairly short period of time. Hunger will return in the following weeks, you may be overeating at this stage. This is why an adjustment is necessary at week 4. Typically, the surgeon or nurse practitioner will add about 1.0 – 1.5 ml of fluid during the first adjustment.

How Adjustments Are Done

Patients worry about getting adjustments, especially getting the first one since there is something about a needle going into your abdomen that frightens them more than the surgery itself. There is nothing to worry about as this procedure is pretty straightforward and typically only requires a single prick of the needle. You may feel a little bit of discomfort when the needle goes in, but the discomfort is no different than getting your blood drawn.

Adjustments are typically done at the office and sometimes may require a trip to the radiology department depending on the method of adjustment the doctor recommends. Before any adjustment is done, a full consultation is required to help the surgeon or nurse practitioner better understand the amount of fluid needed. After the consultation, a proper volume for adjustment will be determined. When doing a traditional adjustment (without the use of X-ray) they will find the access port by having you lay down with a pillow under your back. This makes it easier to find the access port. Some surgeons prefer radiological adjustments which require you to swallow barium and have an X-ray done to while adjusting the band. They will look at the barium flow while adjusting the band. Once there is only a narrow column of barium passing through, the band fluid has been adjusted to the correct level. Then, the needle is removed which concludes your lap-band adjustment session.

There is no right or wrong volume for the fill and should not be compared to other individuals. The fill volume is just a number and is different for everyone. Just because your friend has a fill of 4.5ml does not mean that a 4.5ml fill is right for you. A simple adjustment itself may take only about 3 minutes. After the adjustments, it may take 2-3 days before you can start enjoying solid foods again as the band needs time to adjust. During this time you may feel the need to switch to soft or liquid foods if solid food is uncomfortable. If after 3 days you have trouble swallowing solid foods, contact your bariatric team to see if the band is overfilled.

When to Get Your Band Adjusted

The lap-band fill volume can be overfilled, underfilled or just right.

When the band is too tight (overfilled) this can create an obstruction, which will make it difficult to swallow solid foods. You may start noticing that you prefer softer foods while avoiding solid foods. Solid foods may have trouble staying down.

Common symptoms reported of an overfill:

❖ Difficulty swallowing
❖ Tightness in the lower chest area
❖ Heartburn
❖ Reflux feeling
❖ Vomiting
❖ Night cough
❖ Preferring soft foods or liquids

If you feel the symptoms above, it may mean that your band is too tight and an adjustment may be required to remove the excess fluid.

The opposite can also happen when the band is underfilled. With an underfilled band, there is less restriction which will cause you to be constantly hungry and looking for food. You may also feel that a small meal does not fill you up anymore and you start gaining weight. If this happens, schedule a visit with your surgeon to get an adjustment to help make the band tighter. Sometimes you may experience these symptoms due to band slippage. It is important that at any time, if you feel that the band is not working for you, visit your bariatric surgeon to see want is needed to be done to get you back on track.

Getting the adjustment just right does take time. You will need to listen to your body and see how it responds to each adjustment. The ideal fill happens when:

- ❖ A small meal satisfies your hunger
- ❖ You do not feel hungry throughout the day
- ❖ You are continually losing weight
- ❖ You have no problems with solid foods.

Keep in mind that proper follow-up is needed to get to this ideal stage. Sometimes the band may lose a very small amount of saline over time and a fill is necessary to compensate for the loss. Other times, you may get pregnant and need additional nutritional support, where the surgeon can remove fluid from the band to help make that happen. The adjustment aspect makes the lap-band a very powerful weight loss tool. No other bariatric surgery is adjustable like the Lap-band.

The 12 simple shortcuts to get the most out of your lap-band

1. Exercise between 30-60 minutes a day

2. Be more active, make choices that force you to burn more calories (take the stairs vs taking the elevator)

3. Eat no more than 3 small meals per day

4. Always leave food on the plate, never finish everything on the plate

5. Eat slowly, enjoy the food.

6. Stop eating as you as you feel satisfied and comfortable, but you could still eat a little more.

7. Chew each bite thoroughly

8. Avoid any liquids that contain calories. (juices, sweetened drinks, soft drinks)

9. Select quality / nutritious foods over calorie-rich foods such as fast food

10. No snacking. Do not eat in between meals.

11. Do not drink liquids while you eat solid foods.

Wait 45 minutes after you take the last bite of your meal before you drink any liquids.

12. Be in contact with your bariatric team and complete all the recommended follow-up appointments. Have at least 1 follow-up every six months or sooner.

By following these 12 simple shortcuts, it will help you get the most out of your lap-band. Remember that the lap-band is only a tool and the results will vary on how well you use that tool. When combined with healthy eating choices and regular exercise, the lap-band can be a very effective tool to help you effectively lose weight.

Chapter 11. Bariatric Friendly Recipe Collection

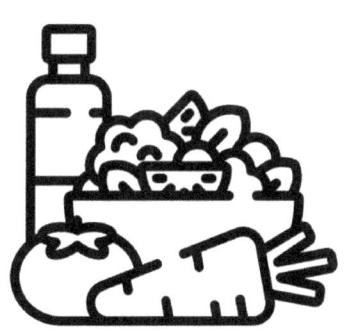

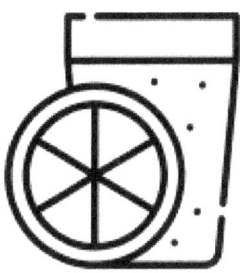

Liquid Diet
Page 127

Puree Diet
Page 143

Soft Foods
Page 163

Solid Foods
Page 187

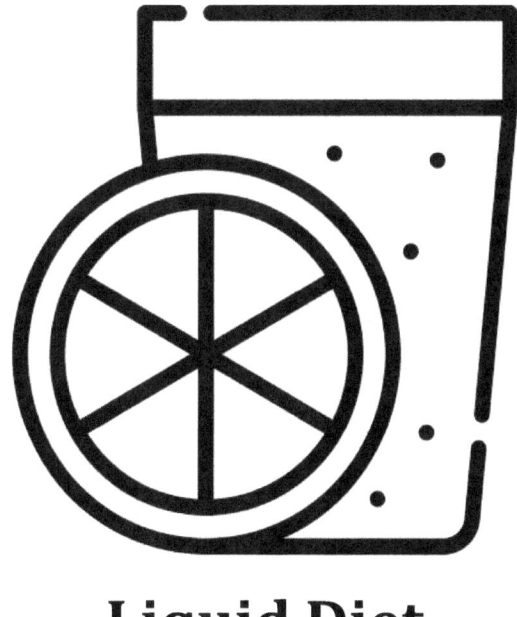

Liquid Diet

Ginger Carrot Juice

Simple juice ready in minutes. Optional: add your favorite protein powder to increase the nutritional value.

Prep:	Yields:
5 minutes	*1 serving*

<u>Ingredients</u>

2 medium carrots, peeled

1 medium apple, cored

1-inch ginger root, peeled and chopped

1 tsp. of lemon or lime juice (optional)

1 package of stevia or no calorie sugar substitute (optional)

<u>Directions</u>

Blend all ingredients until smooth. Strain the mixture through a fine sieve strainer to separate large fiber from the juice.

Chocolatein

Inspired by Mexican style hot chocolate, this recipe utilizes chocolate flavored protein powder for a lower fat content. You can replace the nonfat milk with almond milk, soy milk, or water.

Prep:	Cook:	Yields:
5 minutes	*10 minutes*	*1 cup*

Ingredients

1 cup of nonfat milk

1 serving scoop of chocolate flavored protein powder of your choice

1 tsp. of vanilla extract

¼ tsp. of cinnamon powder

1/16 tsp. of ground cayenne pepper (optional)

Directions

1. In a small pot, warm 1 cup of nonfat milk for 5 minutes or until simmering (make sure not to scorch the milk). Lower the heat.

2. Add cinnamon powder, vanilla extract, ground

cayenne pepper, and chocolate whey protein powder. Mix well.

3.   Cook the mixture for one minute. Remove from heat and transfer to a cup.

Blood Orange Sports Drink

This rehydrating drink is simple to make. You can substitute the blood orange with different fruits such as pineapple, watermelon, strawberry, or mango. The possibilities are endless! Just don't forget to strain the pulps and seeds for a smoother consistency.

Prep:	*Yields:*
10 minutes	*2 servings*

Ingredients

2 cups of coconut water

1 medium blood orange, squeezed

1 tbsp. of honey or 1 packet of stevia sugar

Pinch of salt

Directions

Combine all ingredients together and mix well.

Ginger Chicken Soup

Healthy and lean homemade chicken broth with ginger, garlic, and lemongrass. The aromatic lemongrass adds freshness to the soup with a hint of spiciness from the ginger. This homemade chicken stock can be refrigerated or frozen to prolong shelf life.

Prep:	Cook:	Yields:
15 minutes	2 hours 30 minutes	6 servings

Prep: 15 mins

Cook: 2 hours 30 mins

Yields: 6 Servings

Ingredients

2 oz. ginger root, peeled

8 cloves of garlic, peeled

2 lbs. bone-in chicken, cleaned

2 large carrots, cleaned and thickly sliced

1 medium onion, quartered

1 stalk of lemongrass, cleaned and halved

8 whole peppercorns

1 bunch of scallion (approx. 5 pieces)

2 quarts of water or more

1 tablespoon of lime juice

salt and pepper to taste

Directions

1. Place the raw chicken into a large pot. Fill up the pot with room temperature water just enough to submerge the whole chicken.

2. Cook the chicken at medium high heat, until the water boils.

3. Remove the chicken. Place the chicken to a large bowl. Wash and the chicken with room temperature / cold water to remove the excess oil and blood. Dump the water.

4. In a clean large pot, place the chicken, add clean water and combine all the ingredients in a pot except the salt. Bring to a boil.

5. Skim the floating foam.

6. Lower the heat. Simmer for about 2 hours until the meat can be easily removed from the bone.

7. Strain vegetables, bones, meats, and spices from the broth.

8. Season broth with salt to taste.

9. Let the broth cool or refrigerate overnight. Skim the fat for a leaner broth.

Watermelon Ice Pops

Now you can enjoy juicy watermelon on a stick. The best of all, it is fast, easy, and kids will love it too!

Prep:	*Yields:*
10 minutes	*4 servings*

Ingredients

2 cups watermelon juice (no sugar added store bought juice or homemade freshly pressed juice)

½ tablespoon lime juice

1 teaspoon honey (optional)

Directions

1. Mix all ingredients together.

2. Carefully transfer mixture to the ice/popsicle mold of your choice. Freeze at least for 4 hours (or until firm).

Sugar-Free Hazelnut Iced Coffee

Creating a sugar-free beverage is now simple and easy. You can use light, medium, or dark roasted coffee. (Optional: Blenderize the ice cubes to create slushy iced coffee).

Prep:	Yields:
5 minutes	1 serving

<u>Ingredients</u>

½ cup of brewed decaf coffee, chilled

1 tbsp. of sugar-free hazelnut syrup

1 cup of nonfat milk or your choice

a handful of Ice cubes

<u>Directions</u>

1.   Combine decaf coffee, sugar-free hazelnut syrup, and nonfat milk. Mix well.

2.   In a tall glass, pour the coffee mixture over ice.

Apple Cider

Impress your guests with this simple homemade apple cider. You will be surprised on how delightful the aroma of cinnamon, star anise, allspice, and apple surrounds your kitchen.

Prep:	Cook:	Yields:
10 minutes	3 hours	4 servings

Ingredients

6 whole gala apples, washed and sliced

1 cinnamon stick

½ star anise

3 whole allspice, crushed

6 cups of water

Directions

1. Combine all the ingredients in a medium sized pot. Bring to a boil. Stir occasionally.

2. Simmer covered over low heat for about 3 hours. Make sure that the apples are soft.

3. Turn off heat. Remove the cinnamon stick, star anise and allspice from the mixture. Mash the apples.

4. Strain the cider for a smoother consistency. Discard the solids. Serve warm or chilled.

Matcha Latte

Matcha, or also known as powdered green tea, is commonly used to make teas or as a natural food flavoring. Matcha latte is simple to make and can be served warm or cold. To serve this latte cold, simply add ice cubes and use cold nonfat milk.

Prep:	Yields:
5 minutes	1 serving

Ingredients

1 teaspoons match powder

1 tablespoon warm water

¾ cup hot nonfat milk

1 serving stevia (or sugar substitutes)

Directions

In a cup, combine matcha powder and warm water. Stir until no lumps remain. Add stevia and milk. Enjoy!

Chai Tea

Chai tea is a combination of spices, milk, and tea. This type of tea is very commonly found in India and many other places around the world. In this non-fat recipe, you can add no calories sugar to sweeten the tea.

Prep:	Cook:	Yields:
15 minutes	*30 minutes*	*2 servings*

Ingredients

½ tbsp. ginger, peeled and diced

¼ tsp ground cardamom

1/8 tsp ground nutmeg

1/8 tsp ground allspice

3 whole cloves, crushed

1 whole star anise

1 cinnamon stick

1 tbsp. vanilla extract

1 cup of non-fat milk

1-2 bags black tea, depending on the strength you desire

1 cup of hot water

Directions

1.   Steep the black tea bags in hot water.

2.   Over medium heat, bring the milk with the rest of ingredients to just before boiling. Make sure not to scorch the milk. Stir occasionally.

3.   Add the black tea to the milk mixture.

4.   Lower the heat and cover the pot with a lid. Simmer over very low heat for 10-15 minutes to let the aromatic compounds infuse well with the milk mixture.

5.   Strain the solids and large spices from the tea mixture. Enjoy warm or over the ice.

Strawberry Iced Tea

Quick and easy iced tea perfect for hot summer days. Try this refreshing sweet and tangy iced tea that can be made within minutes. Budget friendly and suitable for the whole family.

Prep:	*Yields:*
10 minutes	*2 servings*

Ingredients

6-10 medium strawberries, chopped

1 tsp lemon juice

2 cups of brewed white tea, chilled

½ - 1 tsp honey or sugar substitute (optional)

Directions

1. Puree the strawberries until smooth consistency.

2. Strain through fine cheesecloth on top of a metal strainer to remove the seeds.

3. Combine the strained strawberry mixture with lemon juice and white tea. Add honey to taste.

Puree Diet

Green Pea Soup

A non-dairy soup that contains protein-rich vegetables. You can use any varieties of frozen or fresh peas such as green, English, snow, and snap peas.

Prep:	*Cook:*	*Yields:*
10 minutes	*20 minutes*	*6 servings*

Ingredients

1 (20 oz.) bag of frozen green peas

4 cups of low-sodium vegetable stock

1 medium onion, chopped

1 clove of garlic, minced

2 leeks, chopped, rinsed thoroughly, and drained

½ cup fresh mint, chopped

½ cup fresh parsley, chopped

1 tbsp. of olive oil

Salt and pepper to taste

<u>Directions</u>

1. In a large saucepan, sauté onion and leeks with 1 tablespoon of olive oil over medium heat for 5 minutes or until tender.

2. Stir in minced garlic. Cook for 1 minute.

3. Add vegetable stock. Bring to boil.

4. Add green peas and cook over medium heat for 3 minutes.

5. Remove from the heat. Add parsley and mint leaves into the peas mixture. Cool mixture at room temperature for 10 minutes.

6. Puree the pea soup mixture in a blender or using immersion/stick blender. Blend until smooth. Add salt and pepper to taste.

Beet Sorbet

This recipe is utilizing an ice cream maker. Be sure to follow the manufacturer's guide to making sorbet. You may try to make this recipe without the ice cream machine, but the texture and the consistency may not be ideal.

Prep:	*Cook:*	*Yields:*
10 minutes	*45 minutes*	*6 servings*

Ingredients

2 large beets, trimmed and brushed

3 tbsp. of stevia

¼ cup of apple cider or apple juice

¼ cup of orange juice

¼ cup of water

1 tbsp. of lemon juice

pinch of salt

Directions

1. Pour just enough water into the cooking pot to submerge the beets.

2. Boil beets for about 45 minutes or until soften in the center.

3. Remove beets from hot water. Set aside until the beets are cool to touch.

4. Clean and peel / remove the skin.

5. Roughly chop the beets.

6. In a blender, combine chopped beets, stevia, apple cider/juice, orange juice, lemon juice, and salt together. Blend until smooth.

7. Transfer the beets mixture into a jar and refrigerate until cold for at least 4 hours.

8. Prepare and process the chilled beets mixture in an ice cream maker - and follow the manufacturer's instruction. Store beet sorbet in the freezer for few hours for a firmer sorbet.

Spiced Eggnog

Bariatric friendly eggnog with nonfat milk. This recipe does not contain eggs or alcohol.

Prep:	Cook:	Yields:
10 minutes	30 minutes	2 servings

Ingredients

2 cups of nonfat milk

3 whole allspice, crushed

2 cardamom pods

3 whole cloves

¼ tsp of ground nutmeg

2 tbsp. of fat-free vanilla pudding

Directions

1. In a small pot, combine all the ingredients over medium heat.

2. Bring to a boil. Stir occasionally. Make sure do not over boil because high heat can scorch the milk.

3. Lower the heat. Simmer covered for 15 minutes.

4.   Remove from the heat and separate the spices with a cheesecloth.

5.   Enjoy warm or iced.

6.   Optional: add vanilla flavored whey protein powder.

Cauliflower Chowder

Heart-warming vegetable soup that's great for the whole family. This recipe is enriched with onion, carrot, garlic, and a hint of nutmeg. Best of all, it is healthy and low in carbs.

Prep:	*Cook:*	*Yields:*
15 minutes	*1 hour*	*6 servings*

Ingredients

1 tbsp. of olive oil

3 cloves of garlic, chopped

1 medium onion, chopped

3 medium carrots, chopped

3 cups of cauliflower, chopped

3 ½ cups of reduced sodium chicken broth

1 cup of fat-free milk

¼ tsp of ground nutmeg

½ tsp of dried basil

1 bay leaf

Salt and pepper to taste

Directions

1. In a large saucepan, sauté garlic and onion with olive oil until soft over low heat.

2. Add the remaining ingredients except the salt and pepper.

3. Bring to boil and let it simmer over low heat for additional 15 minutes.

4. Season the soup with salt and pepper.

5. Remove from heat. Blend the soup/chowder until smooth.

6. Bring it back to boil until the chowder is thickened. Stir occasionally. Remove from heat.

Green Booster Juice

Healthy and refreshing green juice is super easy to make. For this recipe, you only need 4 ingredients; mango, cucumber, romaine lettuce and kiwi.

Prep:	Yields:
5 minutes	1 serving

Ingredients

1 cup of mango, peeled and cubes

1 head of baby romaine lettuce, chopped

1 kiwi fruit, peeled and diced

1 cucumber, peeled and diced

Directions

1. Combine all ingredients in a blender. Blend until smooth.

2. Strain the juice through a fine strainer or cheesecloth if desired.

Virgin Mary Mocktail

A new twist on the Bloody Mary without the alcohol. This simple mocktail contains tomatoes and lime/lemon juice.

Prep:	Yields:
10 minutes	*2 servings*

Ingredients

1 celery stick including the leaves

1 cup of tomatoes, diced

dash of salt

1/3 tsp Worcestershire sauce

½ tsp hot sauce or Tabasco

1 tsp lime juice or lemon juice

1 clove shallot or garlic, minced

1 ½ cup of ice cubes

Directions

1. Blend all ingredients together until smooth.

2. Strain the juice for smoother consistency.

Homemade Applesauce

Versatile made from scratch applesauce that can be enjoyed warm or chilled. Store in airtight glass containers such as Mason jars or canning jars.

Prep:	Cook:	Yields:
15 minutes	*45 minutes*	*3 cups*

Ingredients

3 pounds of apples (about 7 apples), peeled, cored, and quartered

1 tsp lemon zest

3 tbsp. lemon juice

1 medium sized (about 3 inches) cinnamon stick

6 tsp sugar substitute

2 cups of water

½ tsp salt

Directions

1. Add ingredients together into a large pot. Bring to boil. Once boiling, lower the heat.

2. Let the apple mixture simmer covered for 30

minutes or until the apples are very tender.

3.   Remove from heat and discard the cinnamon stick.

4.   Blend the cooked apples until smooth with an immersion blender.

5.   Bring the applesauce to a boil and reduce to the desired thickness.

6.   Remove from the heat.

7.   Storage: Put the applesauce in jars or any glass container with a tight seal. Refrigerate after use.

Strawberry Banana Protein Ice Pops

Easy to follow instructions to make protein-enriched ice pops. This recipe is using premade clear protein drink. For creamier popsicles, you can substitute clear protein drink with 1 serving of vanilla whey protein powder + 1 cup of water/nonfat milk.

Prep:	*Yields:*
10 minutes	*4 servings*

Ingredients

2 cups of fresh/frozen strawberries, washed and stem removed

1 medium ripe banana, peeled and sliced

1 cup of pre-made clear protein drinks of your choice

Directions

1. In a blender, blenderize strawberries until smooth.

2. Strain strawberry puree with a fine sieve strainer or cheesecloth to remove seeds.

3. Pour the strawberry puree back in a blender.

4.	Add the remaining ingredients. Blend until smooth.

5.	Divide the mixture equally in ice pops mold.

6.	Freeze overnight.

Tropical Smoothie

A tropical combination of papaya, yogurt, and banana.

Prep:	*Yields:*
10 minutes	*1 serving*

Ingredients

½ cup of water or nonfat milk

¼ cup of nonfat yogurt

½ medium ripe banana, peeled and sliced

2 oz. ripe papaya, peeled, seeded, and chopped

a handful ice cubes

Directions

In a blender, blend all ingredients until smooth.

Pumpkin Soup

You can create this soup by using oven-roasted pumpkin or store-bought unsweetened pumpkin puree.

Prep:	*Cook:*	*Yields:*
15 minutes	*40 minutes*	*6 servings*

Ingredients

1 tbsp. of olive oil

1 medium onion, chopped

4 cloves of garlic, minced

1 tbsp. of ground cumin

1 tsp of chili powder

½ tsp of ground black pepper

2 cups of broth (chicken or vegetables)

1 can (16 oz) of pumpkin purée – or roasted pumpkin (cut into 3 inches cubes).

Directions

1. In a large pot: sauté onion, garlic, cumin, chili and pepper with olive oil until soft.

2. Add pumpkin puree and broth into the pot. Cook

over medium heat for 5-10 minutes. Stir occasionally.

3. Lower the heat and simmer for 25-30 minutes. Optional: use a stick blender to smoothen the consistency (be careful, it's hot!).

French Onion Soup

Caramelizing the onions is the key to a fantastic French onion soup. Cook over medium to low heat when caramelizing the onion to avoid the burnt flavor.

Prep:	Cook:	Yields:
15 minutes	45 minutes	4 servings

<u>Ingredients</u>

1 tbsp. olive oil

2 medium red or yellow onions, peeled and thinly sliced

1 leek, cleaned and thinly sliced

3 ½ cups of beef stock

2 cloves of garlic, minced

¼ tsp thyme

1 tsp of Worcestershire sauce

salt and pepper to taste

1 tbsp. shredded cheese

Directions

1. In a medium pot, sauté onions and leeks until tender with olive oil over low-medium heat. Make sure not to burn the onion and leek.

2. Stir in the garlic.

3. Add the beef stock and bring to boil.

4. Reduce heat. Cover and simmer for 30 minutes.

5. Turn off the heat and blend the soup.

6. Sprinkle shredded cheese for garnish.

7. Add salt and pepper to taste.

Soft Foods

Cauliflower Risotto

Vegetable risotto recipe without the rice. You can add 3 oz. of diced mushrooms of your choice for additional protein content. This dish is a perfect substitute for a rice-free meal and can be enjoyed with lean proteins such as cooked chicken breast, turkey or salmon.

Prep:	*Cook:*	*Yields:*
15 minutes	*25 minutes*	*4 servings*

Ingredients

1 head of medium cauliflower, rinsed, cleaned, and stem removed

½ medium onion, chopped

3 cloves of garlic, minced

1 tbsp. of olive oil

¾ cup of low-fat milk

½ cup of low-fat cottage cheese

salt and pepper to taste

Directions

1. Cut cauliflower into large chunks.

2. In a food processor, pulse cauliflower pieces to

create rice texture. Set aside.

3. In a medium saucepan, sauté garlic and onion with olive oil for 2 minutes or until fragrant.

4. Add chopped cauliflower and milk. Reduce the heat and simmer (uncovered) for 10 minutes or until cauliflower is soft and fully cooked. Stir occasionally.

5. Combine cottage cheese and continue cooking until the cheese melts. Season to taste with salt and pepper.

Tofu Meatballs

Classic tofu meatballs mixed with mushrooms. This dish can be utilized as components in vegetarian spaghetti marinara or as meat substitution in many soup recipes.

Prep:	Cook:	Yields:
20 minutes	35 minutes	6 servings

Ingredients

1 pack of firm tofu, drained

1 tbsp. of olive oil or sesame oil

3 oz. of mushrooms (Shiitake, Portobello, Cremini), rinsed and cleaned, stem removed, coarsely chopped

½ small onion, chopped

1 garlic clove, minced

¾ cup of panko breadcrumbs

1 ½ tbsp. of low-sodium soy sauce

1/8 tsp. of ground black pepper

1/16 tsp. of red pepper flakes (optional)

Directions

1. Preheat oven to 375F.

2. Line a large baking sheet with silicone baking liner or parchment paper.

3. In a large bowl, mash tofu until smooth or resembles ground beef consistency.

4. Add the remaining ingredients. Mix well.

5. Shape the tofu mixture into small 1-inch balls.

6. Place the tofu meatballs on the baking sheet, and bake for 25- 30 minutes or until golden brown. Turn tofu meatballs over halfway through baking time.

Italian Meatloaf

Family sized sirloin meatloaf with delicious glaze. This recipe comes with two different variations of glaze/sauce. For an easier recipe, you may use store bought low sugar marinara sauce.

Prep:	Cook:	Yields:
20 minutes	1 hour	10 servings

Ingredients

for the meatloaf:

2 tbsp. of olive oil

1 medium onion, diced

3 cloves of garlic, minced

1 large red pepper, diced

1 lb. of ground sirloin

¼ cup of oatmeal

1/3 cup of bread crumbs or panko bread

¾ cup grated hard cheese such as Parmagiano Reggiano

2 eggs

1 tbsp. of Worcestershire sauce

1 tbsp. of balsamic vinegar

2 tbsp. of fresh basil leaves, chopped

1 tbsp. of fresh parsley leaves, chopped

for the glaze/sauce:

½ cup marinara sauce

-OR *MADE FROM SCRATCH VERSION-*

1/2 cup of ketchup

1 tsp of ground cumin

¼ tsp of Worcestershire sauce

¼ tsp of hot sauce/ tabasco

1 tbsp of honey

Directions

To Make the Meatloaf:

1. Preheat oven to 350 degrees.

2. In a medium sized pan, sauté onion, pepper and garlic with olive oil over medium heat. Cook until the vegetables are soft.

3. Remove from heat. Let it cool for few minutes.

4. Combine the remaining ingredients.

5.   Shape the mixture into a loaf on a pre-oiled or parchment paper-lined baking sheet.

6.   Bake for 45 - 55 minutes or until the inner temperature reaches 155 degrees.

7.   Spread the marinara sauce or homemade glaze sauce on top of the meatloaf. Place back in the oven to for 10 minutes.

8.   Allow the fully cooked meatloaf to rest for about 5 minutes.

To Make Homemade Glaze:

Combine cumin, ketchup, honey, hot sauce, and Worcestershire sauce together. Mix well to even consistency.

Turkey Meatballs Soup

Turkey meatballs are great substitutes to regular beef meatballs as they are lower in calories per serving. Seasoned with basil leaves, garlic, pepper, and parmesan cheese give embodied flavors that marries well with chicken broth. You can make the meatballs a day in advanced and keep them in the freezer. You may substitute ground turkey with lean ground chicken if desired.

Prep:	*Cook:*	*Yields:*
30 minutes	*45 minutes*	*8 servings*

Ingredients

For Turkey Meatballs

1 lb of lean ground turkey

1 egg

½ cup of grated parmesan cheese

2 tbsp of fresh basil, chopped

2 garlic cloves, minced

3/4 tsp of salt

1/4 tsp of ground black pepper

For the Broth

8 cups of low-sodium chicken broth

1 cup of carrots, peeled and sliced

1 cup of celery, sliced

¼ bunch of parsley leaves, chopped

1/2 medium onion, chopped

Directions

1. Combine egg, turkey, Parmesan cheese, garlic, basil, salt and pepper in medium sized bowl.

2. Shape the turkey mixture by hand into meatballs. Place shaped meatballs on baking sheet or plate. Let them chill for 30 minutes.

3. While waiting for the meatballs to chill, bring chicken broth to boil, add carrots, celery, and onions. Reduce the heat and let it simmer semi-uncovered for 10 minutes.

4. Add the chilled turkey meatballs. Simmer for another 10-15 minutes. Make sure the meatballs are

cooked thoroughly.

5. Stir in the parsley leaves.

6. Season with salt and pepper to taste.

Tuna Chili

A smarter way to incorporate tuna into your daily meals.
This recipe contains protein, vegetables, and is low in fat.
Hearty meal with lower calories than traditional high fat
and high carbs beef chili.

Prep:	Cook:	Yields:
15 minutes	*35 minutes*	*4 servings*

Ingredients

1 tbsp. of olive oil

1 medium onion, chopped

1 can of tuna (7 oz.) in water, drained

1/2 can of gluten- free beans (7 oz.), drained

1/2 can of tomatoes (7 oz.), chopped

1 tsp of dried chili flakes or to taste

1/2 cilantro bunch, chopped

salt and pepper to taste

Directions

1. Heat 1 tablespoon of olive oil in a medium pot. Add onion and cook over medium-low heat until soft.

2. Add drained tuna, tomatoes, beans and chili flakes.

3. Cover the pot and simmer for about 15 minutes or until the tomatoes soften.

4. Season with salt and pepper.

5. Serve with chopped cilantro as garnish.

Steamed Egg Custard

Soft and silky simple egg custard that only requires two main ingredients. You can mix in cooked chicken, mushroom, or spinach for a more filling meal.

Prep:	Cook:	Yields:
5 minutes	15 minutes	2 servings

Ingredients

2 eggs

¾ cup of water, nonfat milk or broth

¼ tsp. of kosher salt

Directions

1. Prepare/Preheat the steamer.

2. In a medium bowl, beat eggs until the yolks and egg whites until fully combined.

3. Add water/nonfat milk / broth and salt into the egg mixture. Whisk for 30 seconds or until slightly foamy.

4. Divide the egg mixture equally into two ramekins/heatproof bowls.

5. Place the ramekins/heatproof bowls filled with egg custard in a steamer. Cook over medium-low heat for 10-12 minutes or until the egg custards are set.

Tofu and Cauliflower Couscous

A vegetarian and lower calorie meal that is packed with protein. You can utilize leftover cauliflower couscous for mashed cauliflower or as one of the ingredients to make mock fried rice.

Prep:	Cook:	Yields:
20 minutes	20 minutes	6 servings

Ingredients

1 head cauliflower, cut into large chunks

1 (12 oz.) pack of firm tofu, strained and cubed

2 tbsp. of sesame or olive oil

¼ cup of low-sodium soy sauce

¼ bunch of scallion, chopped

2 cloves of garlic, minced

2 tbsp. of mirin (optional)

Salt and pepper to taste

Directions

To Make Cauliflower Couscous

1. Rinse and trim cauliflower's leaves and stem.

2. In a food processor, pulse cauliflower until the cauliflower resembles couscous.

3. In a large nonstick skillet, Sauté raw cauliflower with 1 tablespoon of sesame/olive oil over medium heat for one minute. Add a pinch of salt and mix well.

4. Lower the heat, cover the skillet with a lid, and continue cooking for 5-10 minutes or until tender. Fluff the cooked cauliflower with fork or spatula and set aside.

To Make Stir-Fry Tofu

1. Coat a large nonstick skillet with one tablespoon of sesame or olive oil.

2. Sauté garlic and tofu for one minute over medium heat.

3. Sprinkle chopped scallions and pour soy sauce over the tofu mixture. Mix the mixture and cook for additional one minute.

4. Season tofu mixture with salt and pepper to taste.

Chicken Mushroom Frittata

Simple oven baked style frittata. For a lower calorie version, you can remove some of the egg yolk from the mixture.

Prep:	Cook:	Yields:
15 minutes	15 minutes	6 servings

Ingredients

1 tbsp. of olive oil

6 eggs

½ cup of low fat cheese

3 tbsp. of diced onion

1/4 cup of cooked chicken sausage

¼ cup of chopped mushroom

Salt and Pepper to taste

Directions

1. Preheat the oven to 350 F.

2. In an oven safe saucepan, sauté onions and mushrooms with olive oil until soft.

3.   In the meantime, whisk the eggs and add cheese to the mixture. Season with a dash of salt and pepper.

4.   Incorporate the mixture with the cooked chicken sausage into the saucepan. Let it cook for few minutes.

5.   Pour the eggs and cheese mixture into the saucepan to cover the rest of the ingredients.

6.   Under medium heat, let the eggs cook for 3-5 minutes before placing inside the oven.

7.   Place the frittata in the oven, bake for 10 minutes or until the eggs are fully cooked.

Slow Cooker Chicken Stew

This chicken stew is ready in four and a half hours. Potatoes are optional for this recipe.

Prep:	Cook:	Yields:
25 minutes	4 hours	6 servings

Ingredients

2 medium potatoes, peeled and cut into chunks (optional)

1 cup of frozen corn, thawed

1 cup of carrots, cut into chunks

¾ cup of celery, chopped

1 medium onion, sliced

2 cloves of garlic, chopped

1 cup of tomatoes, diced

1 ½ tsp of ground cumin

1 tsp of chili powder

½ tsp of ground pepper

1 lb. of boneless chicken breasts, cubed

2 ½ of cups chicken broth

Fresh cilantro, chopped (optional) as garnish

Directions

1. Spray a slow cooker with cooking spray.

2. Add potatoes, corn, carrots, celery, onion and garlic into the slow cooker. Stir in tomatoes, cumin, chili powder and pepper.

3. Place chicken on top of vegetable mixture.

4. Pour broth over ingredients. Cover and cook on High heat setting for about 4 hours.

5. Garnish with cilantro if desired.

Omelet in a Cup

An alternative breakfast omelet for your busy lifestyle. Fast and easy! Add cooked lean proteins such as diced chicken breast and peas to increase the nutritional value.

Prep:	Cook:	Yields:
5 minutes	1-2 minutes	1 serving

Ingredients

1 large egg

1 tbsp. of water

Pinch of salt and pepper

Cooking spray

Directions

1. Lightly coat a microwave-safe cup with cooking spray.

2. In a cup, beat egg, water, pinch of salt and pepper with a fork. Mix well.

3. Cook in a microwave for 60 seconds or until egg is fully cooked.

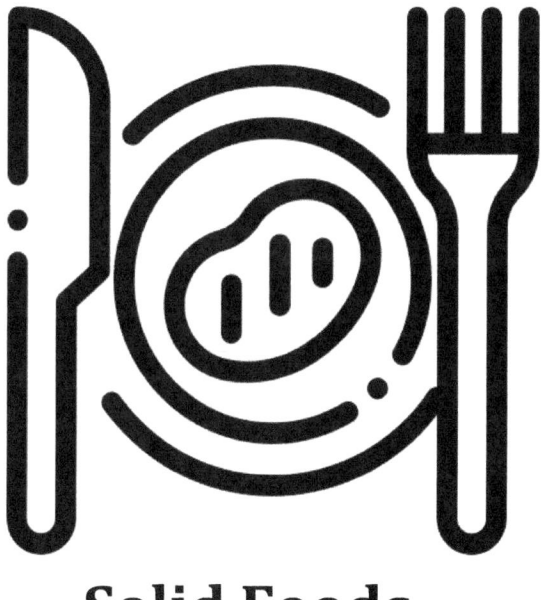

Solid Foods

Oven-Baked Salmon

French style salmon dish that can be ready in less than an hour. Perfect for breakfast, lunch, or dinner. This dish pairs well with cauliflower risotto, spaghetti squash, or salad.

Prep:	*Cook:*	*Yields:*
15 minutes	*25 minutes*	*4 servings*

Ingredients

2 (6 oz.) salmon fillets, deboned

2 sprigs fresh rosemary (or a pinch of ground rosemary)

1 lemon, thinly sliced

1 tbsp. of Dijon mustard

1 tbsp. of olive oil

1/16 tsp. of ground pepper

Directions

1. Preheat oven to 400F. While waiting for the oven to preheat, coat salmon fillets with olive oil and Dijon mustard. Sprinkle, evenly, ground black pepper on each fillet. Place the coated salmon fillets into a shallow baking dish.

2. Cover the surface of the fillets with lemon slices, and top with rosemary sprigs.

3. Bake the seasoned salmon for 15-25 minutes or until fish is fully cooked in the center.

Kale Chips

Crunchy and crispy vegetable chips. Lightly seasoned with garlic, onion, paprika, and dash of salt & pepper. Best of all, it's low in calories per servings!

Prep:	Cook:	Yields:
15 minutes	25 minutes	2 servings

Ingredients

½ bunch of kale leaves, stem removed, washed, and thoroughly dried

1 tbsp. of olive oil

1 tsp. of garlic powder

½ tsp. of onion powder

¼ tsp. of paprika powder

1/16 tsp. of salt

1/16 tsp. of ground black pepper

Directions

1. Preheat oven to 275F. Line a large baking sheet with a silicone baking liner or parchment paper.

2. Tear or cut the kale leaves into large pieces.

3. In a large bowl, toss and combine all ingredients together with hands or tongs.

4. Place a single layer of the seasoned kale onto the baking sheets. Bake kale chips for 20-25 minutes or until crispy.

Baked Orange Chicken

An appetizing orange chicken dish without the excessive oil from deep frying. For faster cooking, you may cut the chicken breasts into smaller pieces (cubed).

Prep:	Cook:	Yields:
20 minutes	50 minutes	4 servings

Ingredients

4 (3 oz.) boneless chicken breasts

3 tbsp. of cornstarch

¼ tsp. of kosher salt

1/8 tsp. of ground black pepper

Pinch of paprika powder (optional)

For The Sauce

½ cup of orange juice

2 tbsp. of brown sugar

3 tbsp. of low sodium soy sauce

½ tsp. of paprika powder

1 tbsp. of cooking vinegar

1 clove of garlic, minced

1 tbsp. of orange zest

4 slices of orange

1 tsp. of sesame seeds (optional)

1 tsp. of cornstarch (optional; to thicken the sauce)

Directions

1.   Preheat oven to 350F

2.   In a medium-sized bowl, combine cornstarch, salt, pepper, and paprika powder. Mix well.

3.   In the same bowl, coat evenly the chicken breasts with the cornstarch mixture.

4.   Bake for 35-40 minutes or until the chicken breasts is fully cooked.

5.   While waiting for the chicken to cook, in a small saucepan, combine orange juice, brown sugar, soy sauce, paprika, vinegar, garlic, orange zest, cornstarch together. Cook over medium heat for 5-10 minutes or until the sauce thickens. Set aside.

6.   When the chicken breasts are fully cooked, lower

the oven temperature to 325F.

7.   Glaze the chicken breasts with orange sauce and place the orange slice on top of each chicken breast. Bake for additional 5 minutes.

Spaghetti Squash

Perfect substitute to the ordinary wheat spaghetti or macaroni. Spaghetti squash is low in calories, carbs and sugars. Makes a great addition as a side dish.

Prep:	Cook:	Yields:
5 minutes	*40 minutes*	*6 servings*

Ingredients

1 medium Spaghetti or Orangetti squash (about 2-3 pounds)

Directions

1. Preheat the oven to 400 F.

2. Slice the squash in half lengthwise from the stem to the tail. Remove any seeds.

3. Place the squash on a baking sheet, cut-side down. Cover loosely with aluminum to minimize over roasting.

4. Cook for 35 - 40 minutes or until the squash flesh

is tender and separate easily.

5. Scrape off the squash with a fork. Gently pull the flesh from the skin and separate into strands to resembles spaghetti. Serve immediately.

Shrimp + Cherry Tomatoes Salad

A simple sautéed shrimp and tomatoes seasoned with garlic, herbs, and a light vinaigrette. You can substitute small shrimp with a larger variety. If so, chop large shrimp into smaller bite size.

Prep:	Cook:	Yields:
15 minutes	*10 minutes*	*2 servings*

Ingredients

1 tbsp. of olive oil

1 clove of garlic, minced

¼ lb. of small shrimp, cleaned, peeled, and deveined

1½-2 cups of cherry tomatoes

2 tbsp. of low-fat feta cheese, crumbled

½ tsp. of dried oregano

¼ tsp. of dried or freshly chopped parsley

1 tbsp. red or white wine vinegar

Salt, pepper, and chili flakes to taste

Directions

1.   In a medium skillet, add a tablespoon of olive oil.

Sauté garlic, oregano, parsley and shrimp over medium heat. Cook shrimp for about 5 minutes or until all shrimp turn pinkish and opaque.

2.   Add cherry tomatoes and wine vinegar. Season with salt, pepper, and chili flakes. Cook for about 1 minute. Once the dish is ready to serve, sprinkle some low-fat feta cheese on top of the salad.

Beef Fajitas

Nutritious Mexican flare dish contains lean beef and vegetables. Pairs well with salsa and cauliflower tortilla. You can substitute sirloin for chicken breast, fish, or tofu.

Prep:	*Cook:*	*Yields:*
15 minutes	*15 minutes*	*6 servings*

<u>Ingredients</u>

12 oz. of trimmed sirloin beef

1 large onion (any varieties), sliced

1 small green bell pepper, sliced

1 small red bell pepper, sliced

1 small yellow bell pepper, sliced

1 tbsp. of olive oil

¼ tsp. of salt

¼ tsp. of ground black pepper

½ tsp. of ground cumin

1 clove of garlic, minced

½ bunch of fresh cilantro, chopped

1 fresh lime, squeezed

1 tsp. of chipotle powder

Directions

1. In a medium bowl, combine salt, pepper, cumin, garlic, and cilantro.

2. In the same bowl, coat evenly the sirloin beef with the marinade mixture.

3. Refrigerate the marinated beef for at least 3 hours.

4. Grill the beef steak over medium heat. Cook for 4-5 minutes on each side or until your desired doneness.

5. Remove the steak from the heat and let it rest.

6. In the meantime, over medium heat, sauté onion and bell peppers with lime juice and olive oil. Cook until the onion and bell peppers slices are tender. It may take about 5-7 minutes.

7. Slice the rested steak to an approximately quarter

inch in thickness.

8.   Combine the sliced steak with the vegetable mixture. Mix well.

Shrimp + Zucchini Noodles

Simple Mediterranean flair dish with a twist. This recipe contains zucchinis that resemble flourless angel hair pasta for a lower calorie meal.

Prep:	Cook:	Yields:
10 minutes	*15 minutes*	*4 servings*

Ingredients

4 medium zucchinis, seeded

1 tbsp. of olive oil

2 cloves of garlic, minced

½ lb. of shrimp, cleaned, peeled, and deveined

¼ cup of chicken or seafood stock

1 large lemon, zested and squeezed (discard the pith and seeds)

½ tsp. of kosher salt

½ tsp. of black pepper

10-12 cups of boiling water to blanch (flash cook) zucchinis

Directions

1. Finely slice zucchini lengthwise to resemble noodle strands.

2. In a large pot filled with boiling water, blanch (flash cook) the zucchinis for 2 minutes. Set aside.

3. Coat a large skillet with one tablespoon of olive oil. Over medium heat, sauté garlic and shrimp. Cook for 3 minutes.

4. Pour chicken or seafood stock over the shrimp and garlic mixture. Cook for 1-2 minutes or until the shrimp are fully cooked (turn pinkish and opaque).

5. Add blanch zucchinis, lemon juice, lemon zests, salt, and black pepper. Mix well. Cook for an additional minute and remove from heat.

Blackened Tilapia

Simple and quick fish recipe. You can substitute Tilapia fillet with Basa, Halibut, Cod, or any white fish.

Prep:	*Cook:*	*Yields:*
10 minutes	15 minutes	2 servings

Ingredients

2 (3 oz.) Tilapia fillet or any white fish

1 tsp. of roasted garlic paste

½ tsp. of ground smoked paprika

1/8 tsp. of chili flakes or chipotle

1/8 tsp. of ground cumin

¼ tsp. of kosher salt

¼ tsp. of ground black pepper

Cooking spray to coat the skillet

Directions

1.   In a small bowl, combine roasted garlic paste, paprika, chili flakes/chipotle, cumin, salt, and pepper together.

2.   Rub the dry rub mixture to the fish liberally.

3. Heat the non-stick skillet lightly coated with cooking spray. When the skillet is hot, place the seasoned fish. Over medium heat, cook for 3 minutes on each side or until cook thoroughly.

Pan-seared Cod Fillet

This is a simple and light dish that does not require complicated ingredients. This versatile fish dish perfectly paired with cauliflower risotto or refreshing balsamic tomato salad. For easier flipping, you can use a non-stick skillet, but in general, other skillets such as cast iron, ceramic, and stainless steel skillet will work.

Prep:	Cook:	Yields:
15 minutes	10 minutes	2 servings

Ingredients

2 (3 oz. each) Atlantic Cod fillet

1 tbsp. of olive oil

1 clove of garlic, minced

2 lemon wedges (about ¼ of lemon each)

1 branch fresh thyme (optional)

1 branch fresh rosemary (optional)

Pinch of salt and black pepper

Directions

1. Season fillet with minced garlic, a pinch of salt and black pepper (optional: sprinkle thyme and

rosemary leaves). In a preheated skillet, add one tablespoon of olive oil.

2.   Place the fish fillets and let it cook for about 2-3 minutes on each side or until fully cooked in the center. Remove fish from heat and serve with lemon wedges if desired.

Balsamic Tomato Salad

Marinated tomato salad that pairs well with grilled chicken, turkey, or fish. You can use cherry, grape, heirloom, or any mix varieties of tomatoes.

Prep:	*Yields:*
10 minutes	*4-6 servings*

Ingredients

Roughly 1 lb. of tomatoes (any varieties of tomatoes), sliced

¾ cup of small/baby part-skim or low-fat mozzarella cheese

2 tbsp. of olive oil

6 tbsp. of balsamic vinegar

½ tsp. of kosher salt

¼ tsp. of black pepper

1 clove of garlic, minced

2 tsp. of dried basil or a small bunch of freshly chopped basil leaves

½ cup of pitted olives

½ cup of pickled onion (optional)

Directions

1. In a bowl, combine and toss all ingredients together.

2. Cover the bowl with plastic wrap or transfer to an airtight container.

3. Store and let the flavor infused together in a refrigerator for at least 2 hours.

References

[1]Bluementhal MD, Susan, and Samara Levin. 2016. *Global Obesity: A GRowing Epidemic.* https://www.huffpost.com/entry/global-obesity-a-growing_b_9139554

[2]National Institute of Diabetes and Digestive and Kidney Diseases. 2017. *Overweight & Obesity Statistics.* 08. https://www.niddk.nih.gov/health-information/health-statistics/overweight-obesity

[3]World Health Organization (WHO). 2018. *Obesity and Overweight.* 02 16. http://www.who.int/en/news-room/fact-sheets/detail/obesity-and-overweight.

[4]World Health Organization. 2017. *Prevalence of obesity among adults, BMI ≥ 30, age-standardized Estimates by country.* http://apps.who.int/gho/data/node.main.A900A?lang=en

[5]Simon, Ben. 2016. *Child obesity an 'exploding nightmare' in developing world: WHO.* 01 25. https://www.yahoo.com/news/child-obesity-exploding-nightmare-developing-world-132206370.html.

[6] Finkelstein, Trogdon, Cohen, and et al. 2009. *Annual Medical Spending Attribute to Obesity*. Health Affairs.

[7]Lakartidningen. 2005. *Sugar triggers our reward-system. Sweets release opiates which stimulates the appetite for sucrose-- insulin can depress it.* 05.
https://www.ncbi.nlm.nih.gov/pubmed/15962882

[8]Harvard School Of Public Health. 2016. *As overweight and obesity increase, so does risk of dying prematurely.* 07 13.
https://www.hsph.harvard.edu/news/press-releases/overweight-obesity-mortality-risk/

[9]Cawley, J, and C Meyerhoefer. 2012. *The medical Care Costs of Obesity: An Instrumental Variables Approach.* Vols. 31(1):219-230. Journal of Health Economics.

[10]Cawley, J, JA Rizzo, and K Hass. 2007. *Occupation-specific Absenteeism Costs Associated with Obesity and Morbid Obesity.* Vols. 49(12):1317-24. Journal of Occupational and Environmental Medicine.

Gates D, Succop P, Brehm B, et al. 2008. *Obesity and presenteeism: The impact of body mass index on workplace productivity.* Vols. 50(1):39-45. J Occ Envir Med

[11]Proc Am Thorac Soc. 2008. *Obesity and Obstructive Sleep Apnea: Pathogenic Mechanisms and Therapeutic Approaches.*
https://www.ncbi.nlm.nih.gov/pmc/articles/PMC264 5252/

[12]Wilkinson MD, Lawrence H., and Ole A. Peloso MD. 1981. *Gastric (Reservoir) Reduction for Morbid Obesity.* 05. https://jamanetwork.com/journals/jamasurgery/article-abstract/587478

[13]Kuzmak, LI. 1986. *Silicone gastric banding: asimple and effective operation for morbid obesity.* Vols. 28:13-8. Contemporary Surgery.

[14]American Society for Metabolic and Bariatric Surgery (ASMBS). 2017. *Public Service Announcement regarding Discontinuation of the Ethicon Endo-Surgery Curved Adjustable Gastric Band (Realize/Swedish/SAGB).* 1 18. https://asmbs.org/articles/psa-curved-adjustable-gastric-band.

[15]Michelson, Robert, Diane K. Murphy, Todd M. Gross, and Scott M. Whitecup. 2013. *LAP-BAND® for Lower BMI: 2-Year results from the Multicenter Pivotal Study.* Vols. 21:1148-1158. Obesity.

Notes

_____

_____

_____

_____

_____

_____

_____

_____

www.ingramcontent.com/pod-product-compliance
Lightning Source LLC
Chambersburg PA
CBHW071255220526
45468CB00001B/135

* 9 7 8 1 7 9 0 5 8 6 1 8 9 *